# THE *handbag* BEAUTY BIBLE

# THE *handbag* BEAUTY BIBLE

Josephine Fairley & Sarah Stacey

With illustrations by
David Downton

KYLE CATHIE LIMITED

# THE *handbag* BEAUTY BIBLE

This is the book you've been telling us you want: the ultimate, slip-it-in-your-handbag guide to the beauty products that really do live up to their promises. So that when you're out shopping, you have all the inside info – on the real beauty steals, blow-the-budget indulgences and the more natural products from the mountain of choice out there.

Throughout the book you'll find our own favourite products – which we've been lucky enough to try during our combined 30-plus years in the beauty business – but what makes our *Beauty Bible* series unique is the fact we test products on real women, and analyse their feedback. Every product is sent to a panel of ten dedicated beauty-hounds – more than 2,400 women in all, recruited through www.beautybible.com – who filled in detailed forms and awarded scores that enable us to pinpoint the products that really work.

We tested products from over 280 brands across 70 categories, making this, we're sure, the biggest-ever independent consumer survey of beauty products ever carried out, worldwide. We know that, against such huge competition, any product that makes it to these pages has seriously impressed our testers. There really are products out there that do the business but no woman we know has the time – or the cash – to try them all. So, with our teams of testers, we've done the homework for you!

For the growing number of wannabe-natural beauties, we have gone

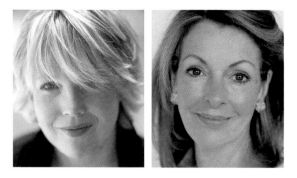

half-blind scanning the lists of ingredients on the back of products. So here is how it works: if a product is 100 per cent natural, then it gets two daisies. If it contains genuinely high levels of botanical ingredients, we award it one daisy. What we don't expect to find anywhere near the top of the ingredients list for those one-daisy products are synthetic or petroleum-based ingredients: we do expect high levels of natural elements – eg, shea or cocoa butter. There are, alas, products that imply they're more natural than they are, and sometimes you'll find items from the same company with a daisy in one category but none in another.

We've also talked to some of the leading experts in the beauty world to gather their time-saving tips for beauty-shopping, and to make-up artists, hair pros and nail gurus for their best beauty secrets.

We hope you have lots of fun shopping for what we're confident are the very best beauty buys. Prices, names and availability were checked at time of going to press – but beauty companies have been known to change or discontinue products without notice.

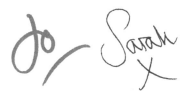

PS Do log on, for our beauty advice, insider info and more: www.beautybible.com

# CONTENTS

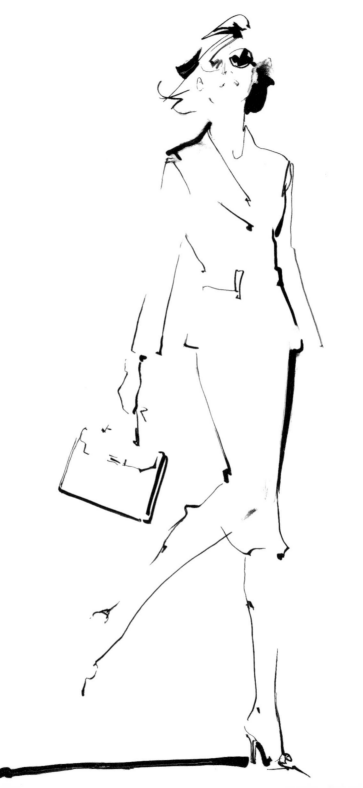

# Shopping

First things first: insider info on
how to shop for beauty products,
from some of the leading beauty
insiders. Whether you're on the
prowl for make-up or nail treats,
skincare or hair products,
read their short cuts
to smart beauty choices!

# Tips for *beauty* shopping

Whether you're off on a spree to stock up on skincare, or dashing in for a quick lipstick fix, beauty shopping is an investment in both money and time. As you know, this book gives you the lowdown on the 'Beauty Oscar'-winning products in 70 categories – helping to steer you towards products that are worth splashing out on – but in a perfect world, a girl's just gotta have fun actually doing the biz, too. So we turned for advice on being a savvy beauty shopper to our friend Lorna McKay, formerly head beauty buyer for Harrods perfumery and cosmetics, and currently consultant for QVC, the shopping channel. Here's what she tells her best friends – and wants the rest of the world to know!

## First things first

● Remember, the customer is queen – so walk like a goddess, never put up with bad service and never be pressured into buying something you're not 100 per cent convinced of. 'I'll think about it' is a good line.

## Essential prepping

● Make sure you know what type of skin, hair and nails you have before you set out. Ask an expert if you don't – a facialist, hair stylist, manicurist can give you the facts.

● List any known sensitivities and, if you know them, the ingredients that cause them – that way, you can check labels and eliminate any likely troublemakers.

● Target your good points so that you can maximise them. So if you've got sensual, full lips, for instance, you'll probably want a wardrobe of lipsticks and glosses, to play them up.

## Make a list

● Know what you want: change of image, new lippie or essential supplies.

● Write down the items you need and the ones you want!

● Set a budget. Resist the temptation to

make impulse buys, unless you have money to burn and unlimited shelf space.

NB: you may find it easier to focus on shopping/styling for one area – skincare, haircare or make-up – at a time, otherwise it can all become overwhelming.

## Decide where to shop

● Big department stores will usually give you the widest choice, and you can always book in for a free makeover with a company you like the look of.

● Alternatively, you might have a dynamite small pharmacy/beauty/hair salon or day spa near you; ask friends where they shop and plan your route.

● Once you have found a knowledgeable, well-trained consultant who doesn't oversell, keep in touch with them. As with a hairdresser, tell them about your lifestyle, budget, beauty routine and the clothes you like so they can help you to look the best you can. But remember: always be honest if you don't like something.

● And if you can't get out and about to shop, remember you can now get almost everything shipped to your door via catalogues, online and TV shopping.

## Handbag helpfuls

● Tissues, cotton buds, moist wipes, magnifying mirror.

● Small empty pots, so you can ask for a sample, if there are no giveaways. Don't be shy about asking for samples: good companies want you to try their products.

● Small notebook, to make your own personal *Beauty Bible* – or scrawl all over this one. We do!

● Minimum make-up – your absolute essentials, in case you have to re-do yours during the trip.

## Organising

● Have a good breakfast first and pop a couple of fruit and nut snack bars and a bottle of water in your bag.

● Shop between Monday and Thursday, early morning if possible, when stores are less busy and consultants have more time and energy.

● It's fun shopping with girlfriends, but if you want special attention, shop alone.

## Try before you buy

● If you're shopping for new make-up, particularly foundation and blusher, go with a clean skin. Would you try a dress on top of another one? We don't think so…

● Ask the consultant for a demo of how best to test/apply.

● Use cotton buds to apply; never put fingers in pots.

## Making the most of freebies

● Free makeovers are always on offer in big stores, sometimes in specialist boutiques, too, though you may need to book ahead.

● Stores often have evening events, with experts on hand and lots of special buys.

● Some companies will even do special evenings for groups of friends.

● Watch out for trial sizes and promotions – they're economical ways of trying products.

● Stock up on products you use regularly at sale time.

**PS** Read this book and make notes before you do anything else!

# Q What do you *really* truly need in your make-up bag?

Most of us lug around heavy bags, stuffed full of products, like a kind of security blanket. But suppose you simply can't do that? Or you just want the basics for your desk drawer? Which items are indispensable?

F or insider advice, we went to make-up expert Jenny Jordan, who told us that you really need only a handful of key items – the make-up basics that will take you looking glossy and gorgeous from breakfast with the boss, or a presentation in front of 500, to dinner with – well, whoever your heart desires. 'It's all about simplicity and grooming. Natural-looking eyes and a glossy, slightly darker or brighter mouth looks pretty, modern and gives you confidence,' says Jenny.

So here's the lowdown on what you need. And the great thing, of course, is that our ten-woman panels of testers have trialled masses in each category to save you time, energy and money finding the best. Plus, having been lucky enough to try almost everything out there ourselves, we tell you throughout this book the products we love, too.

## Foundation

To find a shade that exactly matches your skin, test above your – pre-moisturised – jawline; the product should disappear straight into your skin. Then apply the foundation – aka base – with your fingers, a sponge or, for preference, a foundation brush, to achieve a flawless finish. Several companies, including Prescriptives and Lancôme, now offer these, as does Jenny.

## Concealer

Choose a pencil to cover spots, a liquid formula to camouflage under-eye shadows, and a cream/stick/wand concealer to cover dark pigmentation, or bruises. Apply after your moisturiser and foundation (if wearing), and blend gently with a clean, small brush.

## Blusher

For the most flattering natural look, opt for a creamy product – or even a cheek tint – in a colour that gives an extra warm glow, rather than being tempted by the extreme of hot red 'painted' cheeks. To blend in colour, dab the tip of a foundation brush on to the pan of colour – or the end of the blusher stick – and stroke smoothly on to your cheekbones, starting from below the outer edge of the eye iris.

## Mascara

Brown for blondes, black for brunettes is the rule; avoid faddy bright colours. Test by rubbing

# A Almost certainly *less* than you have in there now!

the mascara between your finger and thumb: choose a creamy, rich, inky formula – it will make lashes look glossy. Avoid the types that dry quickly and look cakey on your fingers – they'll look the same on lashes.

## Brow pencil

Choose a soft shade that matches your natural brow colour. Apply after foundation and powder, lay a sharpened pencil flat against brows and make small strokes, applying as little pressure as possible, then brush out using a clean mascara wand. Finish with Tweezerman brow mousse.

## Lip balm

Waxy, creamy-textured balms last and last; natural-based fragrances taste less chemical. Apply ten minutes before lipstick. Or, for a long-lasting creamy finish, apply lip pencil all over the mouth after balm.

## Lip gloss

Look for a non-sticky, sheeny product in a flatteringly natural (-ish) shade. Apply to lower lips and pinch together, then use lip pencil to give fuller look.

## Lip pencil

It's helpful to have two pencils: a light natural one for day, and a slightly darker one for evenings. Storing them in the fridge will help them to last longer on your lips. Sheeny, shimmery pencils have the advantage of looking subtle, and you can just sketch in the lip edge without it looking fake.

## Lipstick

Opt for sheer, creamy, glistening products, rather than the dense, matt ones – they will look much more youthful, natural and pretty, once applied. Brush on lipstick with a lip brush, and outline with pencil to even up the lips; blot, then, for longer-lasting colour, reapply the lipstick.

**And for lipstick colour?** Try the following: the rule of thumb is that if three people give you a compliment, then you should stick to that colour!

● **Blondes** with cool-toned eyes – grey/blue – and skin should opt for the more muted pinky tones. (If you're 'cool', you probably don't tan easily.)

● **Brunettes** with dark eyes and fairish skin should go for apricots, goldy peaches and rosy caramels; those with olive skins should choose brown with a hint of red; if you have deeper caramel skin, opt for sheer bricky rust; black skins – amethyst or mauve, with glisten.

● **Redheads** with very fair skin and blue/grey eyes suit cool beigey apricot.

● **Grey/silver/white hair** and fair skin suits hot pink; more sallow skin, rosy pink.

# Is your *make-up* past its use-by date?

You wouldn't dream of eating food that's gone past its 'sell by' date – but you might well still be trying to eke out a Jurassic Age mascara

So, how can you tell if cosmetics have gone off? In a nutshell, rely on your eyes, nose and common sense: if you perceive changes, bin the product. The only exception is eye make-up removers containing camomile, which can go from bright blue to dingy grey in a matter of weeks. This is a natural breakdown and not harmful; it can be avoided simply by keeping the product in the bathroom cabinet. Generally, though, how long should things last? Here's our lowdown…

**Mascara:** buy a new one at least every six months – and before that, if it goes lumpy or changes texture. Remember, don't ever lend your mascara to anyone – it's a quick way to spread an infection.

**Eye make-up:** powder shadows, cream shadows and pencils should last for years, but if you do suffer an eye infection at any point, get rid of what you were using at that time in order to avoid reinfection. Liquid eyeliners should be replaced as often as mascaras – and again, neither a borrower nor a lender be.

**Foundations:** these are designed to last for between one and two years, but if they're exposed to light and changes of temperature, the oils can start to go rancid and separate before that.

**Blushers:** powder blushes are good almost for ever – bugs can't breed in the dry formula – but cream blushers should be replaced every year, at a minimum.

**Nail varnish:** this should last for a year, but if it goes lumpy before that, get rid of it – it'll lead to a less-than-perfect manicure, anyway, with blobbiness and bubbling. NB: supermodels keep theirs in the fridge.

**Fragrance:** again, your nose will tell you if it's in perfect condition, although it should last at least a year – and sometimes much longer. Fragrance can start to smell less than sexy if it's exposed to sunlight, so it's best to keep it in the dark, or – better still – the fridge. This can be very bracing! It's also nice to tuck scent in your lingerie drawer.

**Eye cream:** this can last up to a year or two, but once again, use your nose; if it seems to smell different, ditch it. Don't leave it where the sun can get to it.

**Moisturiser:** unopened, this can last two or three years, but up to six months if you're using it. Bin it if the smell or consistency changes. Can be kept at room temperature, or in the fridge. Likewise cleansers and toners, which should never be diluted.

**Sunscreen:** this is one product that it's crucial to replace this every year. That may seem expensive, but the screening ingredients can lose their potency if they overwinter in your bathroom cabinet, exposing you to the risk of sunburn next summer.

 *tips*

● Keep cosmetics and skincare away from light and heat. Lots of beauty editors store theirs in the fridge.

● Travel with cosmetics in your hand luggage, to avoid exposing them to extremes of temperature in the aircraft hold.

● Use the spatulas and nozzle caps which come with products; they're designed to stop you contaminating the ingredients with less-than-spotless fingers. Q-tips® are useful too.

● Clean spatulas often with hot water, then dry them on cotton wool – a grubby spatula's no better than a finger.

● Look for pump-action products – they stop air/germs getting in.

● Never water down cosmetics, as you change the precise balance of preservatives added to keep a product safe.

● Keep wide-mouthed jars firmly screwed.

● Always wash and dry your hands before applying skincare or make-up.

● Keep your make-up brushes standing in a jar with the bristles upwards, suggests New York make-up artist Mollie Roncal. And every two weeks, wash the bristles with baby shampoo, followed by conditioner to make them nice and soft.

# Shop for your *hair type*

Here's a little secret: even hairdressers are bewildered by the ocean of products designed to keep your crowning glory looking gorgeous. So we asked superstylist Kerry Warn of John Frieda, who tends Nicole Kidman's tresses, to cut a path through the mop jungle

Most bathrooms are full of products that were always irrelevant and are long past their use-by date, says Kerry. The reason? We're not honest with ourselves about exactly what our hair's like, so we can't give it what it really needs. 'Work with your hair type and you'll make life a lot easier,' says Kerry. So, three things: talk to your hairdresser about the nature and condition of your hair, the type of products he/she suggests, and how to use them to maximum advantage. Then – and this is crucial – read the labels before you buy, and, at home, follow the instructions to the letter.

## Hair basics for everyone

- **Shampoo and conditioner:** choose products for your hair type – the labels are a strong clue! So, moisturising/volumising for fine/coloured/dry hair, and so on.
- **Wide-tooth comb:** to comb through conditioners and treatments.
- **Tail or fine tooth comb:** for styling and distributing products evenly through hair.
- **Brush:** to give your mane a good brush before and between shampooing.
- **Hairdrier:** worth looking for a professional/salon one if you have lots of hair.

## haircare tips

- Most knots are at the back, so brush from the base of the scalp, and work forwards.
- Chemically treated hair tends to be more tangled.
- Never brush wet hair: you may damage it.
- Apply a treatment or conditioner to a section at a time – from the back – working through with your fingers. Then comb right through.
- With any product, start at the back with a very small amount – less is almost always more.

## For fine flat hair

- **Volumising/bodifying spray (or mousse)**
- **Vent brush**
- **Hairspray**

Every woman with this type of hair wants body, but don't overload it with product. A good cut every four to six weeks is vital; then use a volumising spray (or mousse). After washing, towel dry, comb through with a wide-tooth comb, then rough-dry – head upside down – with a hairdrier, before applying. Target where you really want the lift – crown, sides or fringe usually – and spray the roots so you don't create a 'helmet'. Use a vent brush to lift as you direct the drier – don't use a diffuser or nozzle – to dry in the product. Finally, mist just the area/s you want to hold with hair spray – avoid spraying all over.

## For frizzy and/or curly hair

- **Masks/oil treatments**
- **Serum**
- **Professional hairdrier with diffuser and nozzle – plus straightening irons, if you like**
- **Natural bristle round brush**
- **Wax**

Regular weekly masks or treatments are essential. After every shampoo, Kerry recommends a good quality serum – but do remember to read the instructions first. He likes to squeeze the moisture out of the hair but not towel dry. Then, sectioning from the back, put a little product in the palms of your hands, rub through hair, and comb with your wide-tooth comb, then the fine one, to help the product glide evenly from root to end. Let hair dry naturally, or blowdry – from the back – with a professional hairdrier fitted with a big, round diffuser, using a natural bristle, round brush. To counteract flyaways – and 'break up' shorter styles – use a very tiny bit of wax, warmed in your palms then distributed through your hair.

## Thicker, straighter hair

- **Masks/oil treatments**
- **Mason Pearson brush, plus natural bristle round brush for blowdrying**
- **Professional hairdrier with diffuser and nozzle – plus straightening irons, if you like**
- **Lightweight serum that can be used on wet and dry hair**
- **Wax**

Always aim to add moisture with shampoo, conditioner and masks. To rehydrate hair after – and between – shampoos, apply a lightweight serum that can be used on wet or dry hair. Remember: dry-textured hair tends to get drier in the winter and coloured hair is even more haystack-like in the summer – so dry, coloured hair needs mega-TLC all year round. Blowdry and style as for frizzy/curly hair.

## accessorising

You can go from day to evening in two minutes max with one or two lovely hair accessories, says Kerry, who likes using pretty vintage slides and combs: 'Nothing too big or glitzy, but just sparkling enough to give a sense of evening – rather than the endless scrunchies or comb clips.' Take some vanity time to play with your hair. And don't feel that DIY is going to be less effective than hours in the salon: 'A gentle, spontaneous look, with a few tendrils escaping can be very beautiful,' says Kerry.

# The how-to guide for

Well-kept hands and feet are as much of a beauty asset as clear skin and glossy hands, but which products do we really need? For the lowdown, we turned to master manicurist Leighton Denny

Few of us have the time or cash for a professional manicure and pedicure every week of our gorgeous lives – so we need to be able to re-create a salon effect at home. Leighton Denny of Urban Retreat, at Harrods, has created picture-perfect looks for dozens of advertising campaigns – not to mention celebrities such as Jade Jagger. He's won the Nail Technician of the Year award so many times, they've given him a gold statue, banned him from entering – to give everyone else a chance – and made him a judge, instead. So, a good chap to give us his nail know-how, then.

## And according to Leighton, this is what you really, really need...

- Hand and cuticle cream
- Cuticle treatment
- Nail oil
- Buffer
- Rubber hoof stick
- Soft grade natural nail file
- Toenail clippers
- Base and top coats
- Nail polish

## How to choose a polish

Polish looks different in the bottle from on the nail, so it's worth testing how sheer or dense the colour is. Take nail polish remover wipes on your shopping trip so you can quickly clean any polish, dirt or fluff off your nails and test the product in store. (See nail polish removers, pages 88-9.) If you're having a professional manicure, ask the manicurist to try out the colours, so you can both decide. Never buy cheap polish: Leighton believes you get what you pay for – and we agree.

## Your most flattering colour

Coffee and toffee shades suit all skin tones. Dark colours look striking on short nails. Avoid salmon pink – it doesn't suit anyone.
- **Fair skinned with blonde hair:** all shades of orange, pink and purple.
- **Fair skinned with dark hair:** all shades of brown.
- **Redheads:** all shades of coral red, brown and bronze.
- **Dark skinned with dark hair:** shades of red and violet.
- **Olive skins:** deep reds, rich browns, dark berry colours and rich roses.

# happy hands
# and fantastic feet

**Brown or black skins:** reds with a blue undertone, deep purples, wine reds, any shade of brown. Soft pinks are flattering, hot pinks fab!

## So you've chosen your shade – now for a perfect finish

**DO** use a base and topcoat to protect and seal in colour, plus a quick-dry product to speed the drying process (it also protects the polish from smudging and prevents clothing and fluff sticking to the polish – see our Tried & Tested quick-dries on pages 86-7 for the testers' favourites).

**DO** give yourself plenty of time for each coat to dry before applying the next layer.

**DON'T** do your nails in a rush. Make sure you have everything you need at hand and then just sit back and relax.

**DON'T** panic if you chip your nail polish. The best chip quick fix is to dab a little nail polish remover on to your fingertip and smooth out the chip. Then paint on another layer of polish.

## Leighton's top tip

'If there was one piece of advice I could give everyone, it would be to use a good nail oil daily. It delivers instant moisture, helping keep nails durable and cuticles healthy.'

## the filing file

**FACT: all nails look better if they're neatly and expertly filed. So, Leighton advises:**

**DO** file fingernails in a shape that mirrors your own cuticle line. It's the most flattering.

**DON'T** use coarse emery boards on fingernails: they can damage the nails, causing them to split or peel.

**DO** choose a soft-grade natural nail file.

**DO** file nails from the outer edge to the centre, but don't 'saw' back and forth because it damages the nail.

**DO** use clippers to cut toenails. Cut them straight across and file from the side to the middle, rounding the corners to help prevent ingrown nails. Ideally, file every day with an emery board.

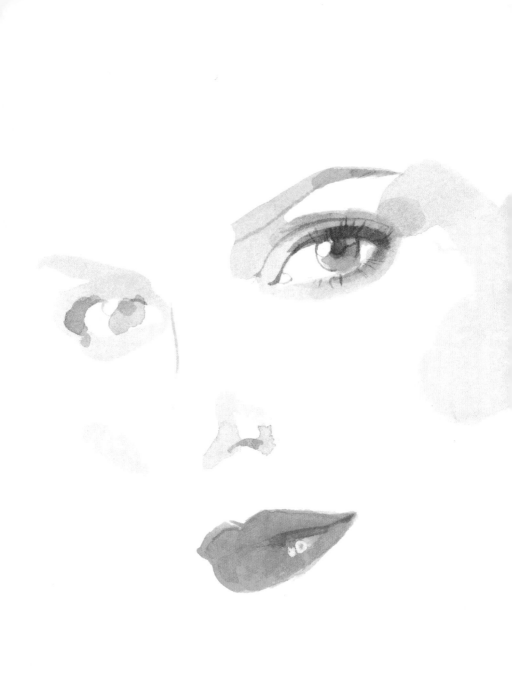

# Make-up

2

We love make-up: the girly glosses, powders and paints that cheer us up – and make us look like a prettier version of ourselves. But what's worth spending on? All is revealed in this chapter

# make-up primers

Suddenly, there's a flurry of make-up primers being launched. Designed to go over moisturiser and under make-up, they might seem yet another extra step in your regime – until you read these reviews by the testers who trialled these top-scoring products, and found themselves universally converted

We asked our ten-woman panels to report on how silky and smooth their skin felt after 'priming', and whether or not the primer helped their make-up to (a) go on more easily and (b) stay put longer. The consensus was that these do both, and – in some cases – more.

## Smashbox Photo Finish Foundation Primer, £30/27.5ml

**Score: 8.45/10**

Smashbox is a Hollywood-based range, sold through shopping channel QVC in the UK, founded by the grandsons of Max Factor. Created for the movie industry to increase the durability of foundation while on the set, it can be used with or without moisturiser underneath.

**Comments:** 'Really magical-textured gel, instantly absorbed, leaving a smooth canvas for make-up; you only need one pump' • 'make-up lasts a full day with no top up; diminished pore size and lines, so overall look was more polished

and smoother' • 'this evened the skin, filling and smoothing small blemishes and irregularities' • 'it has to be the most amazing beauty "find" in a long time' • 'my mother, who is 66, uses it on the backs of her hands, giving them a smooth, matt finish – invisible but beautifying'.

## Bobbi Brown Vitamin Enriched Face Base, £32/50ml

**Score: 8.4/10**

Scented with geranium and grapefruit oil and enriched with vitamins A, C and E, this lightweight balm is designed for all skintypes and is one of Bobbi's own faves. 'It smooths the skin, ensures make-up glides on perfectly and smells amazing,' she tells us. It scored only just behind Smashbox.

**Comments:** 'Real bonus for a busy woman: left skin feeling like silk; make-up went on like a dream, minimised pores, leaving an almost porcelain finish' • 'several people said how lovely and radiant my complexion looks when I use this' • 'made my make-up look much more professional' • 'absolutely fabulous; make-up felt fresh at the end of the day – great moisturiser'.

## Estée Lauder Spotlight Skintone Perfector, £23/50ml

Score: 8/10

This features 'micro-prism technology', which preps skin for smooth make-up application and bounces light off the face. Our testers were impressed by the radiance-enhancing ability, which comes from mulberry extract. With antioxidant vitamins C and E, Lauder promise it also works to fade age spots within three to four months.

**Comments:** 'Great for covering uneven or crinkly-looking skin and wrinkles; gives an iridescent glow to skin' • 'really evens skin tone' • 'took away all the red' • 'enhanced my features, with or without foundation' • 'this was an excellent base for make-up – I felt radiant'.

## MAC Prep & Prime Skin, £16/30ml

Score: 7.95/10

This brand new launch from the make-up artists' brand is packed with silicones that create a velvety 'canvas' for make-up. MAC also claims it calms, soothes and lightly hydrates the skin, as well as blotting excess oil and reducing redness.

**Comments:** 'Great base for make-up; slightly shimmery so gave a nice healthy glow' • 'I liked the handy dispenser pump' • 'gel-like cream that melted in to skin and left it like velvet with a slight dewy glisten' • 'gave a flawless finish to make-up'.

## M&S Autograph Illusions Revitalising Moisture Base, £13/20 ml

Score: 7.3/10

M&S say that using this affordable primer will allow for a fresher, less mask-like application of make-up and brighten skin with an ultra-fine shimmer – in short, 'perfect, photo-shop skin'.

**Comments:** 'Satiny, soft and cool on skin; sank in very quickly; striking difference to evenness of skin tone' • 'don't have to retouch powder on oily

**WE LOVE…**

Having trialled it for this book, Jo is totally converted to Origins A Perfect World (below), 'which really does help my make-up stay put longer. I use it every morning and look forward to the citrussy scent.' Sarah doesn't bother with primers – yet – but always leaves ten minutes between applying moisturiser and putting on foundation – otherwise your 'face' is liable to have disappeared by lunch time.

areas as much' • 'gave skin a bloom I hadn't seen in ages' • 'irons out blemishes and has a light-diffusing glow that looked great in photos'.

## Origins A Perfect World White Tea Skin Guardian, £26.50/30ml

Score: 7.2/10

The most natural of the primers that scored well, this earned rave reviews for its mimosa, lemon, orange and bergamot fragrance, as well as its performance. It's packed with antioxidant white tea, plus walnut extract, magnesium, vitamin E and dimethicone, a silicone derivative, for silky skin.

**Comments:** 'Make-up looked fantastic, stayed put and looked fresh for hours' • 'lovely to use, sank in easily, enhanced radiance' • 'foundation looked really good, more radiant, soft and dewy; women who haven't tried this don't know what they're missing; the only present I ever want'.

# skin brighteners

Brighteners work by giving the complexion an instant boost: rather like primers, they go over moisturiser to create a base for make-up – but usually deliver an extra element of illumination, in the form of light-reflecting particles that can 'blur' lines

**tip** When you're looking tired and/or low, send the blood whooshing to your head by standing with your feet a hip-width apart and gently lowering your head as near the floor as you can, hands resting below your head, each on the opposite elbow. Stay there for a few moments, breathing deeply and slowly. Come up very gradually, uncurling your spine, then stretch your arms to the ceiling and out to the side. For an instant glow, pinch your cheeks or tap them firmly.

Skin brighteners are great for perking up skin that's dull or basically looks as exhausted as you feel, helping to create the illusion of more luminous skin. They're particularly good under evening make-up. If you want a super-matt complexion, these aren't for you – but if you're after a little extra dewiness, a little extra glow, you'll want the following lowdowns from our testers. NB: the only high-scoring budget buy in this category from Nivea, which featured in our last book, has been discontinued, alas.

**Top Treat** Chanel Précision Maximum Radiance Cream, £39/50ml

**Score: 8.3/10**
Prettily and freshly scented, this apricot-tinted, lightweight, luxury cream scored extremely well – and almost all the testers said they'd invest in it after trialling. Chanel prescribe a specific massage technique – outlined in their leaflet – to further enhance the cream's glow-getting effect. It is designed to have anti-ageing benefits – improving skin texture, cell renewal and microcirculation – but our

testers were assessing the short-term I-want-gorgeous-skin-*now* effect.

**Comments:** 'When I first tested this, my baby was three weeks old and I looked pale and tired, but after using it I looked refreshed and alive – absolutely amazing! The baby is now nine weeks old and I am very tired, but with this cream, I glow. I love it!' • 'skin looked healthier and moisturised, felt very soft and supple – and radiance was increased' • 'lots of comments from friends about how healthy I look' • 'the glow from this lasted all day – I even received compliments about my complexion'.

## ☀ Aveda Tourmaline Charged Radiance Fluid, £30/30ml
### Score: 8.25/10

A lightweight gel, packed with antioxidants, including green leaf tea and vitamin C, this also incorporates bio-fermented yeast, corn-derived sugar and clary sage, to help refine skin by encouraging its natural ability to shed complexion-dulling dead cells. It is said to work over the longer-term to reduce wrinkles – but for this trial, our testers were asked to assess its power to improve radiance instantly, which is another of Aveda's claims.

**Comments:** 'Makes skin look like I've been for a brisk walk by the beach – love the fragrance, typically Aveda – woody, mossy, natural' • 'lovely product to use, particularly during the winter months, when skin can look quite grey' • 'skin looked glowing – with or without foundation'.

## Guerlain Divinora Pure Radiance, £35/30ml
### Score: 7.93/10

True luxury, this: reflective particles of real 24-carat gold are suspended in a clear gel, to

make skin look radiant. Guerlain claim Pure Radiance can work as a moisturiser, too – it has vitamin E and hyaluronic acid in it – or it can be layered on over your regular cream.

**Comments:** 'Blended beautifully for a glowing, even-toned, long-lasting and flattering finish' • 'skin definitely looked more radiant' • 'definite radiant glow, with golden sheen – slightly glittery' • 'my face appeared more youthful, with a subtle, shimmery glow; I liked the all-over softness this gave to my face'.

# mattifying products

Women usually want to shine in our careers, good works, even amateur dramatics – but not, we've found, our T-zones! Hail, then, to a new generation of products targeted at oily and shiny skin, to keep skin matt and velvety all day long

This category includes mattifying moisturisers as well as oil-absorbers that are designed to be applied over or under make-up. We chose specifically oily- and complexion-skinned testers for this trial, and we're sorry to report that there were no winners worthy of a daisy for naturalness, or a 'Beauty Steal' tag; if you want truly matt skin, it seems you'll have to splash out. There's no 'We Love' for this category: luckily, we don't shine very often – dryness is our problem.

## Clarins Instant Shine Control Gel, £15/200ml

*Top Treat*

### Score: 8.31/10

This, Clarins tell us, is 'a unique combination of transparent oil-free gel and matt powders', which allows skin to breathe while the formula combats shine in two ways. Pure silica microspheres form an ultra-sheer, non-pore-blocking film on the surface – which continuously absorbs oil – while the gel mixes with the skin's natural sebaceous secretions to alter their reflective properties, so skin appears matt. They recommend using it over day cream and under make-up on forehead, nose and chin, and suggest that during the day – especially in hot climates – it can also be dotted over make-up, as needed. Testers found it took time, both practising and between putting on product and make-up.

**Comments:** 'The best product I've ever found for my very oily skin: usually my skin is shiny within two hours; this time there was still no shine after five hours – a minor miracle! But powder formulations tended to cling to it' • 'lovely gel to use; no downside for me; made my skin very smooth and matt – shall recommend it to my very oily-skinned daughter' • 'liked the lightly perfumed Clarins French smell' • 'this had an immediate mattifying effect'.

## Molton Brown Instant Matte Shine Control, £25/30ml

### Score: 8/10

From the British brand recently snapped up by Japan's Kao Corporation – who now also own John Frieda – comes this oil-free mattifying fluid to be applied each morning to clean skin. The oil-controlling ingredients are Russian larch tree mushroom extract and desert chapparal – and there's a chemical SPF15 sun filter, in the form of ethylhexyl methoxycinnamate, to protect against UVA/UVB rays. Testers found that the pump action could be hard work.

**Comments:** 'Easy-to-follow instructions; skin looked immediately matt and very smooth, though it needed moisturising later' • 'nice product and worked well; will use when I'm working – as a beauty consultant – and applying a full make-up' • 'very good light moisturiser; significantly reduces the size of pores for much smoother and less shiny skin' • 'creamy lotion set to a very dry matt finish, made a really good base and foundation, set quite well, and definitely lasted longer; might try using on eyelids to stop the shiny effect on them' • 'gets rid of oiliness without drying my skin; make-up didn't look caked on – will also use it without any make-up for hot-weather oiliness'.

## Estée Lauder Clear Difference Advanced Oil-Control Hydrator, £23/50ml
**Score: 7.72/10**

This is a light moisturiser with mattifying properties, thanks to a blend of oil-controlling powders, micro-sponges and something that Lauder call Absorbex™ Complex, which they claim helps actively re-programme skin over time so that it produces measurably less oil. Skin-calming caffeine and sucrose also feature, and Lauder recommend using it morning and evening, after cleansing.

**Comments:** 'Genuinely delighted with this; I've tried many, and this is the first that does what it says on the tin' • 'easily and quickly absorbed, long lasting, and great for touch-ups' • 'excellent as a base' • 'wonderfully smooth and shine-free skin, which is a miracle' • 'very luxurious, and solved my main beauty problem – a shiny nose and chin' • 'at 22, my skin is prone to acne and

 One reason noses get oily so fast in summer – and even break out – is sunglasses! Oil builds up on the nose-piece, so rinse off the oil and bacteria every few days, and dry thoroughly.

congestion – this helped significantly, levelled out oily areas, and my skin felt clean and fresh'.

## Shiseido Pureness Mattifying Stick, £15/15ml
**Score: 7.7/10**

This convenient stick – which is packaged in a 'cool and sexy' metallic casing – is swiped over skin, swiftly absorbing excess sebum and helping to camouflage pores so that they appear less obvious. It's part of a wide range of Pureness products to feature the brand's special sebum-absorbing technology, targeted at young, problem skins – but useful for oily complexions of all ages, we'd say.

**Comments:** 'Simple instructions tell you to use after cleansing, toning and moisturising: just apply on areas with open pores and smooth in; turns from very smooth and creamy to powdery dry on face – made my skin smooth and flawless' • 'loved the fact it's an immediate fix – I felt like the longer I used it, the fewer open pores I had' • 'found that my shiny areas didn't look shiny any more' • 'useful to combat shininess and open pores on the chin, nose, between eyebrows and on patches of forehead' • 'I'm sceptical of "magic" products normally, but I was amazed at this and immediately recommended it to two people' • 'so quick and easy to use'.

# all-in-one compact

For women with too much to do in too little time,
these are a godsend: go-anywhere compacts of creamy base,
which cover a multitude of sins and don't need powdering

These can be applied with a damp sponge, for extra coverage, or a dry one, for light coverage or to 'blot' shine – there's usually a sponge in the compact. Testers were asked to comment on coverage, finish and whether or not the product was drying – which can be the only downside of these time-savers. No 'natural' contender scored well enough with our panellists to be featured here.

### Shiseido The Makeup Compact Foundation, £27

**Top Treat**

Score: 8.77/10

Shiseido recommend that this creamy foundation is best for oily skins requiring maximum coverage with a light, matt finish. Created with the input of make-up artist Tom Pecheux, it features a 'Prismatic Powder',

to bounce light off the face and deliver flawlessness, with the bonus of an SPF15. In ten shades.

**Comments:** 'Best ever – very natural yet covered everything' • 'lasted better than many – seven to eight hours' • 'a lovely dewy feel' • 'I especially liked the fact that this smart compact could be refilled'.

### Prescriptives Liquid Touch Compact Makeup, £25

Score: 8.08/10

This incorporates skin-caring ingredients – wheat protein complex, collagen-stimulating polypeptides and antioxidants – in a lightweight foundation, to hydrate and soothe skin while evening out its tone. We seriously approve of the fact this comes in a wide range of shades – 15 in all.

**Comments:** 'It blended seamlessly for a dewy, scrumptious finish; very light

# foundations

and moisturising but covered thread veins, open pores and blemishes; very long lasting' • 'beautiful foundation: covering yet translucent; literally 'melts' into skin, leaving it radiant, glowing and youthful' • 'probably the best foundation I've ever tried'.

## Guerlain Divinora Teint Expert Confort SPF15, £29.50

**Score: 7.95/10**

Guerlain subtitle this 'Exquisitely Fine Powder Foundation Compact', and rhapsodise: 'like the soft caress of a veil of silk, it sheaths the skin with an incredibly matt finish.' The compact certainly has a high glam factor; some loved the hefty gold refillable compact, some found it was a little too 'ritzy looking' but most agreed that the formulation itself – in four shades – delivered great results.

**Comments:** 'Glides on easily with a damp sponge' • 'divine smell – light and sexy' • 'very easy to build coverage to disguise veins and my red cheeks' • 'natural dewy finish' • 'I'd been dying to try an expensive foundation and this far exceeded expectations' • 'good staying power'.

## Chanel Teint Compact Crème Universel SPF15, £26

**Score: 7.95/10**

This creamy, fresh-feeling foundation, which Chanel bill as 'a vitamin fresh cream make-up', comes in a mirror-less screw-top jar – with sponge, rather than a palette – and boasts a moisturiser and a dry oil in the formula, to leave

skin supple. They advise applying with a dry sponge only. Choose from six shade options.

**Comments:** 'Probably the best foundation I have tried – didn't need reapplication but when tested, smoothed on nicely' • 'very sheer; made my skin look flawless' • 'glides on; blended like a dream' • 'the one foundation that looks natural on me'.

## *Beauty Steal* Revlon New Complexion One-Step Compact Makeup, £9.99

**Score: 7.87**

Offering what Revlon describe as 'medium' cover which is 'buildable', this oil-free, one-step foundation offers a choice of six shades, with an SPF15. Be aware, though: any SPF in a foundation works only where you've applied it!

**Comments:** 'A dream to use' • 'went on easily, didn't clog pores and left skin looking smooth and moisturised' • 'didn't irritate or look heavy, and would be great for dull winter complexions that need a boost' • 'coverage even and flattering'.

# stick foundations

We love stick foundations because they double as time-saving concealer and base, in one twist-up, go-anywhere product. Just apply a touch extra where required on spots, blemishes or broken veins

*tip* Bobbi Brown recommends having a 'wardrobe' of three shades of foundation: one for everyday use, a darker shade for summer, and a lighter shade that can double as a concealer. 'The idea is to mix any combination of the three, anytime you need,' she says – so you always have the perfect colour for skin, winter or summer. Remember to dot on very lightly with your ring finger or a damp sponge and build up coverage gradually, rather than slapping it on – otherwise you'll get the pancake look.

Our testers were not greatly convinced by many of the stick foundations they tried, and only two of the dozen or so sampled really made the grade with them, as you will see here. And there are no Beauty Steals or products with daisies for naturalness in this section, because they just didn't score highly enough. We admit that testing foundations for our *Beauty Bible* books is logistically challenging. Our approach is to put together a panel of women with similar skintones, then send the same shade to all of them; we specifically ask our testers to ignore how well – or badly – the shade matches their skin, and focus their reports instead on coverage, ease of use, texture, and so on. Please remember that the key to choosing a good foundation is taking time to test as many as you can, so you arrive at a perfect match with your individual skintone.

## Top Treat
### Shiseido Stick Foundation SPF15, £25
**Score: 7.2/10**

Offering moderate-to-maximum coverage 'with a dewy, luminous finish', Shiseido promise this stylish product 'pairs naturally with the skin's texture for a flawless finish, while minimising the appearance of pores, fine lines, dryness – and providing exceptional wear'. Now for what our testers thought…

**Comments:** 'Very easy to apply with fingers or a damp sponge; I thought it would be thick and block my pores: completely wrong – it looked very natural' • 'offers good coverage but is non-clogging – also non-drying; actually creamy and almost moist' • 'looked amazing; silky velvety texture I hadn't come across before' • 'once I got it right, it was easier and quicker to apply than my usual liquid brands' • 'huge thanks for this: portable, clean and super easy for touch ups at work and out' • 'doubles as a concealer and has an SPF15, so you need fewer products' • 'I would term the coverage medium but it could easily appear sheerer by applying less and blending it well; the finish is quite dewy, and natural sheen of skin is still evident through it' • 'camouflaged thread veins, open pores and small blemishes' • 'great product that I'll definitely keep in my handbag' • 'very luxurious packaging; didn't need to reapply, but if a small blemish showed through I put a little dab on it' • 'changed my views on stick foundations: a very natural look – like myself, but more polished'.

## Becca Stick Foundation SPF30+, £29
**Score: 6.77/10**

A creamy, non-powder formulation that's suitable for most skintypes, this provides 'sheer-to-medium, natural-looking coverage, giving the illusion of perfect skin', Becca tell us. It's recommended less as a stand-alone product – except for those who want full maximum coverage – more for bits of the face that need camouflage, alongside a liquid foundation or tinted moisturiser. Formulated in sun-drenched Australia, it also offers an SPF30+, and the huge plus-point of Becca's foundations is the incredibly wide shade range on offer: 28 in all, including many formulated for Asian and black skins.

**Comments:** 'Colour (Banana) was one of the best I've found; more of a winter foundation, as it gives very full, smooth, even coverage and feels nice and moisturising; it worked best in areas where I need extra help, with a lighter liquid foundation on other areas' • 'certainly didn't need an extra concealer, which got rid of worries about finding the right shade; very handy to carry round, and liked the high SPF' • 'impressed with how smoothly this went on; it was relatively easy to blend and didn't feel like a mask' • 'nice sleek packaging'.

**WE LOVE…**

We both think you can't beat Bobbi Brown Foundation Stick, £24: Bobbi introduced us to the idea of these portable bases, which she produces in a wide selection of flattering, yellow-toned shades – including Jo's choice, Warm Sand – which help neutralise any redness in skin.

# concealers

Where would we be without concealer? A great concealer is the equivalent of a fairy godmother's wand, magicking away flaws – think broken veins, dark circles, spots – and abracadabra: your skin looks perfect. Our testers trialled absolutely loads of new launches in this ever-expanding category, before reaching the conclusion that some of the classic products on the market are still the best

**WE LOVE...**

We're both huge fans of YSL Touche Eclat (this page), as well as Christian Dior Skinflash, £19, a miracle worker on dark circles. Jo's new fave rave is Champneys' All-In-One Complete Eye Care, £10 (from Sainsbury's only), a cooling, lightweight gel with SPF10, UVA sunscreens and antioxidants, which both conceals and treats.

*Top Treat* **Yves Saint Laurent Touche Eclat Radiant Touch, £21**
Score: 9.33/10

This all-time beauty classic, found in every supermodel and make-up artist's kit, works by 'bouncing' light off the face, creating the optical illusion of flawlessness. The brush dispenser can be stroked along fine lines, to 'blur' them (through light-reflective technology). Our testers report that dark circles really do vanish.

**Comments:** 'Brilliant, especially on frown line and nose-to-mouth laugh lines' • 'really gives oomph to your complexion' • 'most amazing! Covered dark circles under eyes that nothing else has been able to do; truly a miracle' • 'a blank canvas to paint your face on – congratulations, YSL!' • 'gorgeous packaging; very easy to reapply on the run'.

## MAC Select Cover-Up, £11
Score: 8.18/10

MAC advise that this slim tube of product can be used under foundation or on its own. It comes in 15 shades – many more than most concealers currently on the market.

**Comments:** 'Made my skin look fresh and had a velvety texture' • 'particularly good for dark circles' • 'a little goes a long way; tube is easy to control' • 'great for eyelids, especially, to help keep make-up on' • 'I've been looking for a product like this for years – now here it is!'.

## Laura Mercier Secret Camouflage, £25

**Score: 8.15/10**

Choose from six palettes, each with two shades to blend and match to your complexion. Ideally, use a small brush to blend on the back of your hand, then apply. This is a favourite of celebs, make-up artists – and our own Beauty Bible panellists.

**Comments:** 'I *loved* it – the most effective concealer I've ever tried' • 'the two colours in the palette made it easy to match skintone and it stayed on well all day' • 'toned down rosy cheeks very well' • 'hid an angry red spot without caking – an impressive concealer'.

## La Prairie Skin Caviar Concealer Foundation SPF15, £95

**Score: 8/10**

This blow-the-budget product is one of the priciest on the market but you do get two products – concealer and foundation – in one jar with mirror and brush. In eight shades and with SPF15, the duo comes packed with skin-caring ingredients that include lavender, green tea, camomile and La Prairie's signature antioxidant-rich Exclusive Cellular Complex.

**Comments:** 'Skin is really radiant, uplifted, glowing – my colleagues comment that I look flawless when I wear this' • 'blended in beautifully – I'm giving it ten-plus' • 'it's one of the best that I've ever used – if you have something to hide, nothing does it better than this'.

##  Jane Iredale Circle/Delete, £23

**Score: 7.62/10**

This 100 per cent natural choice is based on mineral pigments, in a base of nourishing jojoba, avocado and vitamin K (to work actively on under-eye circles). Three 'duos' are available for skintones from fair to darker. The Circle/Delete 2 option in light and medium peach is said to be

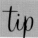

Many women try to eliminate a tired look by using concealer on dark circles, but overlook an important zone: the blue/grey shadow on the inside of the nose bone. Dotting and smoothing concealer there takes off five years – and makes you look as if you had a great night's sleep, even if you were partying till dawn.

especially good for neutralising post-surgery bruising, as well as bluey dark circles. Jane Iredale recommends custom-blending shades with a brush on the back of your hand.

**Comments:** 'Blended well and gave a natural finish – love the fact there are two shades you combine to create a perfect third' • 'light enough to use on bare skin' • 'I used this the morning after a late, boozy night so it had its work cut out – but definitely made me look better, covering all flaws' • 'made a huge red angry spot invisible'.

## *Beauty Steal* Bourjois d'Un Coup de Pinceau Light-Reflecting Concealer, £6.50

**Score: 7/10**

The highest-scorer of the budget ranges we trialled, this streamlined brush-style product comes in a choice of three shades, with added vitamin E, for skin-smoothing.

**Comments:** 'Very light and easy to use – went on silkily, disguised shadows' • 'I still prefer Touche Eclat, but this is a close second' • 'with this and a little powder on top, I was confident without foundation' • 'great for disguising fine lines and dark circles' • 'definitely concealed dark circles and improved the overall look of my eyes'.

# cream blushers

With the right cream blusher, you're not much more than a swipe away from a natural, rosy glow – and no risk of the Pocahontas 'striped' cheek effect a powder blusher may deliver. Here, then, is the crème of the cream blushers

The art of using cream blusher is to apply the teensiest amount and blend outwards. Unlike powder blushers, they work best on well-moisturised (bare) skin, but can also be applied over foundation, and even powder, using fingers – still our favourite make-up tool. As Rebecca Morrice-Williams, whose Becca Crème Blush scored well here, explains: 'A cream appears more real than a powder because the rosy glow seems as if it comes from within, rather than look like it's sitting on top – so you appear younger and fresher.' We asked the brands for universally flattering shades, so, if you're not sure which to choose, those listed here are a short-cut to a natural look.

## WE LOVE...

In Jo's make-up bag, you'll find Becca Crème Blush – in the shade Byzantine that our testers trialled – as well as Laura Mercier Illuminating Stick in Golden Rose Glow, £28, a shimmering rosy shade that she uses when she wants a 'just got back from a blustery walk' flush. Sarah likes Stila's Convertible Colour in the shade Lillium, £17, which 'converts' for lips, too.

### Top Treat

### Pout Flush Blush, £20
**Score: 8.4/10**

A twist-up stick of blusher in *faux* lace packaging, this is as feminine as you'd expect from the ultra-girly beauty brand, which started in a gorgeous boutique in London's Covent Garden and has now gone global. Four shades include Wild Berries, which our testers trialled.

**Comments:** 'Glides straight on with its twist-tube application, very easy; light and smooth yet creamy on skin, pretty natural rose glow through the day' • 'so easy to achieve the rosy-cheeked open-air look; packaging was very pretty' • 'a real joy to use; lovely sheer matt colour – long lasting'.

## Stila Rouge Pots, £13

**Score: 8.06/10**

Packaged as cutely as most of Stila's make-up range, these come in the form of a teensy pot of light-as-air whipped mousse, available in six shades – including Water Lily, a pinky-nude, which our testers trialled.

**Comments:** 'Really lovely! Let my natural skin colour and sheen come through; fantastic light, moussy texture; perfect for a natural look' • 'lovely fresh look, great on clean skin or with foundation, great for young skin, brill if you have slightly hairy or downy skin' • 'can build up colour easily – any mistakes can be blended out in a flash' • 'gorgeous, smooth, silky – not at all greasy' • 'the first blusher that looked natural'.

## Becca Crème Blush, £18

**Score: 8/10**

'Perfectly round-shaped, micronised pigments allow colour to glide on the skin, achieving the most natural-looking colour ever,' claim Becca. Our testers – who tried a shade called Byzantine – agreed. But it should be added that they said the same about our other winners, too.

**Comments:** 'Fantastic product – my skin colour and texture changed using this; made my face look more youthful and healthy' • 'very delicate shimmery finish; gave a youthful effect without being glittery at all' • 'very natural finish, despite my doubts when I first saw the very intense orange shade' • 'very easy to work into the skin and blend across the cheek' • 'liked the classy packaging and little mirror in the lid'.

## Clinique Blushwear, £12.50

**Score: 7.62/10**

Clinique somewhat ambitiously promises 'a healthy angelic glow' with this silky formula, which is a cream-to-powder formulation that 'sets', for

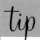

At a pinch, you can use lipstick like a cream blusher – the key to avoiding a doll-like dot of colour is to apply a touch to the end of your fingers, rather than to the cheek itself, pat on to skin, then blend.

'fade-proof, colour-true coverage'. Our testers' shade was Natural Blush – one of three.

**Comments:** 'I really enjoy using it: fingertip application was a breeze; a real natural blush, great for no-make-up look' • 'I loved the shade, and prefer finish to a powder because it looks more natural and less ageing' • 'blends brilliantly; smooth matt finish, more like a cream powder' • 'gave a really natural look with a slight sheen'.

## M&S Autograph Cheek Colourwash, £10

**Score: 7.4/10**

Not exactly bargain-basement priced, but the most reasonable of the high-scoring products here – this light, almost moussy blusher from M&S's most upmarket make-up range comes in a sleek, mirrored, frosted-glass and metal oval-shaped compact. Our testers were sent 'Natural', one of seven Colourwashes available.

**Comments:** 'Gave a natural fresh-air look; didn't need to reapply at work – a touch-up before going out was enough' • 'soft sheer matt finish and natural long-lasting colour' • 'a dream to blend' • 'easy to apply with fingers' • 'smart packaging, went on well, subtle colour' • 'never bought M&S make-up before – this was a revelation; glides on and blends in so easily, perfect colour'.

# cheek tints

Cheek tints, also called cheek stains, can deliver a subtle veil of sheer natural colour, as if you've just got back from a blustery walk. But if you choose the wrong product, you can end up just with clown dots of red on your cheeks that dry before there's time to blend. Find out which tints converted our blushing *Beauty Bible* testers…

Cheek stains are great over moisturised skin (if it's up to scrutiny) for a barely made-up look. Or they can be blended over foundation for a natural-looking glow – but they're not for anyone who likes a full face of make-up, as one tester commented, or for those with high colour, broken veins or rosacea. Once on the skin, they 'set' – making them a budge-proof alternative that lasts all day. But there's the rub, literally: the perfect cheek stain doesn't 'set' too fast, so you have plenty of time to blend it in. Origins pioneered this category with Pinch Your Cheeks, which still performs well, but there are now lots more cheek stains on the market and performance varies hugely. None of the really inexpensive cheek stains tested scored well enough to be included. And, a tip: they do stain – so wash your hands after applying.

### Philosophy The Supernatural Lip and Cheek Tint, £13/6.5ml

**Score: 8.6/10**

The wand-style applicator makes for easy application of this lightweight gel, which is available in three shades and can additionally be used to 'stain' lips (it's flavoured with pomegranate). The colour is 'build-able': you can always layer on more, if desired, to deepen the flush.

**Comments:** 'I look healthy and glow-y, but not too rosy, and it lasts all day' • 'pretty girly packaging: wet consistency blended easily for a very natural flushed finish with no streakiness' • 'makes me look younger!' • 'adore the finish, colour, smell and consistency' • 'no powder-like residue'.

### Bliss Ink Pink Blushing Balm, £18/14g

**Score: 8.35/10**

Like most cheek stains, this gel looks rather scarily dark while still in the tube but (according to

Bliss), 'the no-fail shade of pink complements any complexion'.

**Comments:** 'Lots of "you look well" comments, which made me *so* very very happy' • 'easy to blend with fingertips' • 'this product has been an absolute godsend: I've looked grey and pasty recently due to morning sickness, but with this even my husband said I looked "blooming" on a particularly sicky morning!' • 'no need to reapply all day – amazing stuff'.

## Pixi Sheer Cheek Gel, £14/10ml
**Score: 8.1/10**

This sheer gel with hydrating, skin-soothing aloe vera comes from the Pixi range created by three make-up artist sisters (one blonde, one brunette and one redhead). It comes in six shades, some with a touch of shimmer; our testers tried 'Natural'.

**Comments:** 'I'm in love with this gel blusher! Makes me look so healthy and cute!' • 'doesn't slip off my oily face' • 'I dab it on my lips and they look like healthy rosebuds' • 'this has got me one hundred per cent hooked – a make-up bag staple' • 'I'm getting compliments about looking fresh-faced and like an English rose' • 'I'm a novice but found it really to use, even on my first attempt'.

## Jelly Pong Pong Jelly Flush, £18/28g
**Score: 7.94/10**

A rather unlikely name for a beauty company, but there you go: Jelly Pong Pong (who manufacture in Italy) say they cater to 'the one-swipe-and-go woman'. This easy-to-use blush is a twist-up stick of jelly-like colour, designed 'to give a natural finish and a dewy tinge with one swipe on the cheeks'. It's available in four shades, each infused with a

 If you still find you have problems blending your cheek stain before it sets, try combining a dash of cheek stain with a 5p-sized squirt of facial serum, advises LA-based make-up artist Troy Jensen.

fruity flavour (melon, peach, grape or cranberry).

**Comments:** 'I used to be a powder-blush gal but I'm so pleased that I persevered: this gives a gorgeous natural rosy glow and I really love it!' • 'went on smoothly and evenly; fresh, natural and dewy-looking – perfect for the more mature lady!' • 'great package appeal: really trendy, my 16-year-old daughter was envious' • 'it's hard to go wrong with this product and it seems like it will last for ever!'

## ☀ Origins Pinch Your Cheeks, £11/3ml
**Score: 7.11/10**

If you are looking for a natural-looking stain that has a slightly more natural ingredient list than most, you could go for Pinch Your Cheeks, a little tube of one-shade-fits-all-skintones super-sheer gel from Origins (one of two 'greener' ranges in the Estée Lauder stable), which comes in a recyclable aluminium tube.

**Comments:** 'I thought I would finish up looking like Coco the Clown but the end result was actually a smooth rosy glow, and very natural' • 'I used it over foundation and it was easy to apply – although you have to make sure you blend it quite quickly' • 'gave a sheer finish that looked like flushed cheeks' • 'there was no patchiness, or any obvious product left sitting on the skin surface'.

# 3-in-1 products

Beauty multi-taskers sound hugely appealing for girls on the run, saving both time and space in our make-up bags. Surprisingly, perhaps, none of the many products we trialled proved universal raves, so the scores aren't that high – but remember that the results are averages of ten testers' scores, so the women who liked them really, really liked them!

These three-in-one products are intended for use on lips, eyes and cheeks: a quick swipe or dab, blend with the fingertips, and – hey, presto! – you're made up. They tend to come in a choice of either pinky or coppery-tan shades, for an instant sun-kissed effect when used alone or over foundation. We asked companies to supply us with shades that would suit all skintones. We haven't included a 'Beauty Steal' in this category because none of the less expensive choices impressed our testers one jot.

*Top Treat*

### Guerlain Terracotta Duo Matt & Shine, £16.50
Score: 7.25/10

This came in quite a long way ahead of the competition: a duo palette with one half sheeny, the other matt. (Both are cream-to-powders, which means they 'set' once you've blended them.) Guerlain's in-house make-up genius Olivier Echaudemaison recommends light touches of the iridescent powder over the arch of the eyebrows and top of the cheekbones, for radiance. In three shades, our testers got to try Duo Dune et Miel, designed to give what Guerlain describes as 'a natural, lightly tanned effect'.

**Comments:** 'Lovely packaging: the matt was great as an eye colour and the shine was lovely on the lips and cheeks. Real bonus to have the three in one' • 'this is absolutely gorgeous, particularly as a blusher; it had a very shimmery glamorous look to it' • 'good to use on the move' • 'I was impressed by the colour and staying power' • 'very useful to glam up your existing make-up for a night out'.

## Clarins Multi-Blush, £13.50

**Score: 6.77/10**

Inside this small red and gold compact, you'll find a lightweight powder-cream containing candelilla wax as well as vitamins A, E and Clarins's exclusive Anti-Pollution Complex. It comes in three glowing shades: rose, chestnut and apricot, which is the shade our testers tried.

**Comments:** 'I loved this product on cheeks, lips and eyes, and it was very long lasting' • 'silky creamy texture goes on like a dream, practically foolproof to apply, and doesn't settle into fine lines' • 'great as a blusher and face shaper, also eye shadow and lip colour – the best thing in my make-up box' • 'sweet little compact, easily carried in a pocket or evening bag'.

## Stila Convertible Color, £17

**Score: 6.55/10**

Make-up artist Jeanine Lobel often used lipstick on cheeks instead of blusher – until she created this creamy, translucent product, which melts into lips, cheeks and eyes and is packaged in a gorgeous embossed aluminium compact. In 12 shades, altogether – and our testers tried Peony, a neutral beige-y pink and one of Stila's bestsellers. Testers liked it for cheeks and lips, but tended not to use it on their eyes.

**Comments:** 'I really loved this product – nice girly packaging, and it made my lips soft and natural alone, or sexy and pouty with clear gloss on top, and great colour on my cheeks. All in all, very sheer and natural looking' • 'wonderful if you are the sort of woman who likes to wear make-up but don't want to look too made up during the day' • 'beautiful, portable packaging and the perfect flushed pinch-your-cheeks

 **Testers tended to say that, while lovely on lips and cheeks, the pinky colour didn't look good on eyes – meaning eyelids. But if you have high brows, as Sarah has, smudging a bit of warm colour on the bone there can have a really flattering effect.**

pink/red – not so good for my eyes!' • 'blended well and stayed on all day' • 'good natural lip colour, best with balm on top'.

## ❊ Origins Sunny Disposition® Bronzing Stick for Eyes, Cheeks and Lips, £15

**Score: 6.33/10**

The choice for wannabe-more-natural beauties, this easy-to-use, twist-up stick is free of oil, talc and aluminium, containing essential oils and floral infusions of cardamom fruit, Roman camomile, lavender and dog rose, to calm the skin. We actually tested this (er, by accident!) twice, and the liquid version of this product – it also comes as a powder – scored more highly as a shimmery bronzer, rather than a three-in-one: you can read those results on page 99.

**Comments:** 'Strange combo that you can use on three areas – I was sceptical at first, until I found that it actually worked. After that I carried it round to use as a booster – extremely handy!' • 'I found it was best used on the areas where the sun would catch your face – particularly cheeks, nose and forehead, to add some shimmer' • 'clean and efficient to apply' • 'this had a lovely gold colour, which was nice and light for my pale skin and blonde hair'.

# cream eyeshadows

Cream eyeshadow is the modern way to wear eyeshadow: it gives a much more natural and flattering effect than powder shadow. Our testers were asked to report on ease of application, blendability, smoothness, the finished effect – and how long the shadow stayed in place

W e asked for neutral colours that would suit most colourings, which in practice meant shades of brown. Two downsides with this type of product: some products tend to crease, so testers were asked to be on the alert for that, and secondly, most are designed to be applied with a (ring) fingertip – and while some testers found that quick and easy, others said it took them a few goes to get right. Even products with a wand applicator, such as Pout Eyeslick (opposite), gave some testers a few fretful moments – the trick, in our experience, is to use a tiny dot, then smudge and blend; they're not intended to be precise and crisp. These factors may account for the relatively low scores overall, from which we've taken the three top-scoring products: we felt to go further down the list wouldn't be useful. There were no natural contenders in this category.

*tip* The best cream shadows gleam, rather than glitter. To test whether a cream shadow is just right – or too 'disco' – make-up guru John Gustafson suggests trying it on your hand. When you turn your hand one way, you should see a sheen, but when you tilt your hand, the colour should look matt. If it's shiny when you tilt your hand in both directions, it's suitable only as a highlighter – for brows.

*Top Treat* **Divinora Soft Colour Cream-to-Powder Eyeshadow, £14**

Score: 7.8/10

The pot alone is seductive: a frosted mini-jar, with a lid of hammered gold: 'very feminine and lovely', said one tester; 'almost decadent', sighed another. But it's the formulation that really wowed them: a light, airy cream, with a blend of polymers and silicones, that transforms to a wisp-of-a-colour ultra-matt finish. Our testers tried Beige Chanvre, a warm taupe, which they liked alone and as a base for other eye make-up. It scored very high marks with eight of our testers, but the average dived because of two who weren't keen.

**Comments:** 'Very easy to apply, light on the eyes and wears like a dream; I'll definitely be buying them for presents' • 'sheer translucent colour that built up really well, giving an elegant sheen; went on smoothly and non-drying, great for more mature skin' • 'fantastic on its own – gives my eyes a glowy, awake, fresh look, and I have received many compliments' • 'a sheeny sort of "my skin but better" effect' • 'I like this as a highlighter under my brow, too' • 'colour and finish lasted for eight hours' • 'this was great for morning make-up – it took away all the blue tones on my eyes in seconds, making them instantly look more human!'

## Pout Eyeslick, £14
**Score: 7.6/10**

The Eyeslicks, in this cult brand's signature girlie packaging, come with a wand, which some testers found helped them dab colour easily and quickly where they wanted – though others said it delivered too much and was messy. The cream is enriched with skin-softening vitamin E, and comes in nine shades. Our testers tried Bee, a warm copper shimmer.

**Comments:** 'Nice slick texture that didn't drag the skin, extremely easy to blend with fingertips' • 'shimmer and smooth; beautiful rich copper-gold colour – more night than daytime' • 'particularly good as a highlighter in the evening, for cheeks, too' • 'lasted well during a couple of Christmas parties' • 'lovely

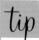

**tip** Olivier Echaudemaison, Guerlain's in-house make-up artist, and the creator of Top Treat in this category, suggests applying a touch of gleaming cream eyeshadow to the inner corner of the eye – the tearduct end – using an eyeliner brush. 'It's especially flattering at night,' he says.

and cool to apply, great for early mornings when your eyes are welded shut!' • 'this was the best of all the ones I've tried: a really nice colour – people asked me where they could get it' • 'I will definitely be buying this again and again; I *loved* it'.

## *Beauty Steal* Almay Bright Eyes Colour Cream Shadow, £5.99
**Score: 7.35/10**

In a choice of four wearable shades (we tested taupey Mocha Shimmer), this lightweight silky formula is hypoallergenic, making it a good choice for anyone with sensitive eyes. It also has special light-diffusing ingredients for a smooth, flawless look.

**Comments:** 'Blended easily to a smooth shimmery (not shiny or glittery) finish; I loved the natural effect' • 'initially I got in a right mess but it became easier with practice, though I think a small applicator would be easier to use than your ring finger' • 'I was very impressed with the results – very shimmery, very pretty; I had quite a few complimentary remarks' • 'lasted all day and when I did re-apply, it didn't cake at all' • 'performed easily as well as its more expensive competitors'.

# mascaras

Some of us love lustrous, thick lashes, while others are after natural-looking definition. But what no one wants is clumping, glooping or flaking. Though mascara is a highly individual preference, the ones here swept the board, hugely impressing our testers. Best of all – as these results prove – fabulous mascaras don't have to break the bank

**WE ♥ LOVE…**

Just as we wouldn't wear the same pair of shoes for every occasion, so we also have mini-wardrobes of mascaras: Dr Hauschka Mascara, £14, for weekends – it's all natural and we love the rose fragrance – Lancôme's ultra-lash-separating Définicils, £17, for everyday, and YSL Luxurious Mascara for the False Lash Effect (opposite) for after dark – the make-up 'LBD'.

 **Max Factor 2000 Calorie Mascara, £7**
Score: 8.56/10

Max Factor promises this 'dramatic look' mascara delivers 200 per cent more volume (hence the 'fattening' name). It's fragrance free and hypoallergenic – so should be good for contact lens wearers – and Max Factor also claim each of the four shades is touch proof, rub proof, smudge proof and snooze proof.

**Comments:** 'Ten out of ten – good for lasting all day' • 'excellent product – value for money and looks fab on' • 'dramatic look and thick, long, glossy lashes' • 'two coats for evening looked dazzling yet not OTT; thick wand but easy to access all lashes' • 'would recommend to anyone – even those with sensitive eyes'.

 **Max Factor More Lashes, £7.95**
Score: 8.4/10

For this mascara (available in four shades), Max Factor tell us they worked with film make-up artists to overcome the problem of clumpy lashes – which certainly never look good on a panoramic cinema screen!

**Comments:** 'I liked that my lashes were more defined but still looked natural' • 'an excellent long-lasting mascara that caused no irritation to my contact lenses – and no smudging either' • 'a well-designed wand which lengthened and thickened evenly' • 'I'm a convert!'

## Biotherm Open Eyes, £11

Score: 8.4/10

Biotherm – a relatively unknown brand, which is actually part of L'Oréal – subtitle this product: 'Endless Lengthening Natural Curve Mascara' – which gives you the general picture. Carnauba and beeswax help spread the pigment from root to tip, while the curling effect is achieved by a combination of rice waxes, applied with a super-separating, patented brush. It's allergy tested and fragrance free, in three shades.

**Comments:** 'The perfect mascara: absolutely no clogginess, clumps, or smudging' • 'this made my lashes long and thick – really opened up the eye area' • 'both lengthening and curling' • 'lovely to use, easy to remove; lengthened and covered but looked very fine' • 'there was no need for an eyelash comb as lashes were nicely separated, with even coverage' • 'I loved the shiny silver container'.

## Yves Saint Laurent Luxurious Mascara for the False Lash Effect, £18

Score: 8.27/10

Despite the va-va-voom full-lash effect that this glamorously packaged product delivers, it is said to be suitable for those with sensitive eyes and contact lens-wearers – and certainly, none of our testers found any bad reactions to report. There are six shades in the range to choose from.

**Comments:** 'This has excellent lengthening properties' • 'it's the best mascara I've used; creates a lovely, long, lustrous look – looked just like false lashes after two coats' • 'has a very user-friendly wand for accessing all lashes; with this, who needs eyelash curlers?'

## ☀ Origins Fringe Benefits, £11

Score: 8.05/10

Origins call this 'lash-loving mascara' because it contains conditioning agents like carnauba wax, camomile and Damascene rose. It was the highest scoring of the more natural products we tried, and comes in black or brown.

**Comments:** 'Nice compact brush; the bristles make it easy to apply for a natural look' • 'this stayed on well; made my lashes look longer and quite natural' • 'this product is good for those who don't need "special effects" such as thickening or curling' • 'this is brilliant for daywear and I certainly found it very natural looking'.

# waterproof mascaras

We challenged our testers to find waterproof mascaras that stay smudge-free during weepy movies, emotional encounters, rainy days, swimming and steamy showers – but which also come off, at the end of the day, without pulling all their lashes out

**WE LOVE...**

Jo is a real waterproof mascara expert, since she swims in the sea from May to November in Hastings. Her long-standing fave is Chanel Drama Lash Extreme Wear Mascara (opposite) – but she now can't decide between that and Clinique Gentle Waterproof Mascara (also opposite), which really is as easy to remove as they promise. Sarah became so fed up with panda eyes out riding that, having lashes that are dark already and being lazy about mascara removal, she gave up wearing any except for days in London and evenings out on the Dorset tiles. Neither of us would ever have our lashes dyed, though, because of the risk of a severe allergic reaction.

Waterproof mascara technology isn't yet perfect, and none of the products scored universally high marks with all ten testers, so the ones on these pages are the best of a mixed bunch. There are no natural contenders in this category, because synthetic ingredients are needed for the 'raincoat'-ing of lashes – but the good news for anyone on a budget is that the highest-scoring product is a 'Beauty Steal'.

*Beauty Steal* **L'Oréal Longitude Waterproof Mascara,** £7.99
Score: 7.88/10

Features L'Oréal's patented Extensel® formula, to 'lengthen lashes by 30 per cent' (so L'Oréal tell us), with a 'high definition' brush, offering more bristles than most. What difference does that make? It apparently improves separation of lashes, while 'stretching' them simultaneously. Available in black only (but we think that's the only colour mascara anyone should wear – even baby blondes).
**Comments:** 'Outstanding product: the real test is when you top up later in the day and it still

looks good' • 'curled lashes upwards attractively – and survived the swimming pool at the Datai Hotel, Langkawi' • 'completely waterproof, even in the pouring rain' • 'I was told three times while wearing this mascara that I had amazing eyes – so I think it's brilliant'.

## Clinique Gentle Waterproof Mascara, £12.50
Score: 7.75/10

A recent launch which impressed most testers because it does, as Clinique claim, 'whisk off easily – no rubbing, tugging, losing lashes'. It also has a particularly well-designed brush, for all-round lash coverage, is available in black and brown, and is said to be suitable for contact lens wearers.
**Comments:** 'I have a tendency to tears – movies, weddings, funerals, songs – so I'd look like a drippy hag if I didn't use waterproof mascara: I've tried numerous ones and this is my favourite' • 'most definitely waterproof – withstood tears, swimming and shower – and you don't have to tug the eye area to remove it' • 'just the right length wand with a decent brush' • 'didn't crumble, flake, clump or smudge' • 'looked really natural with two coats' • 'absolutely fine with contact lenses'.

## Chanel Drama Lash Extreme Wear Mascara, £16
Score: 7.2/10

Like the Clinique winner, this has a thick, surprisingly chunky brush, to coat lashes from root to tip with no clumping. Drama Lash is based on natural waxes, pro-vitamin B5 and ceramides, to condition lashes, while the waterproofing action is down to 'organic syrupy polymers and mineral waxes', they tell us; Drama Lash comes in four shades.
**Comments:** 'Good wand, and lashes looked lovely and natural; I tried it in the rain, in a steamy

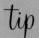 **'Dual-phase' eye make-up removers are best for removing waterproof mascara – see our reviews on pages 48-9 – but also try the 'rolling' technique: dunk a Q-Tip in remover, then gently roll it over the lashes. It should whisk away any bits a cotton pad has left behind. But never, ever rub.**

bathroom and crying, then tried to remove it with water and an ordinary cleanser – it simply wouldn't budge' • 'stayed in place while swimming, but was easy to remove with eye-make-up remover' • 'very good, lustrous results' • 'lashes are longer, glossier'.

## Estée Lauder Illusionist Waterproof Maximum Curling Mascara, £16.50
Score: 6.94/10

Estée Lauder's popular curling mascara is now available in a waterproof formulation, and in four shades. According to Lauder, it plunders technologies from the aerospace and textile industries: inspired by NASA research, 'Illusionist blends spheres of air gels into a curling polymer matrix'. Be that as it may, it received somewhat mixed reviews: some loved it, and some weren't so sure, but we still feel it worthy of inclusion in a tough category.
**Comments:** 'I'm not a lover of waterproof mascara but this was one of the best I have tried' • 'a fantastic mascara – no clumping on lashes and the brush seemed to be loaded with just the right amount of product each time' • 'I found it to be totally waterproof – in the shower, the gym, cycling on a windy day'.

# brow pencils &

Ask any make-up artist: brows 'frame' the eye – and when you get your brow shape and shade right, you may find you need less make-up altogether. Our testers were assigned the palest shades available in each range of brow beautifiers, because it's a common mistake to go too dark, says make-up artist Sonia Kashuk: 'If you have brown eyebrows, grey-brown is better than dark brown – and blondes can use taupe.' So now you know

**tip**
Jo swears by make-up pro Karen Mason's advice to use two shades of brow pencil for her fair brows: a pale taupey base with a slightly darker shade stroked gently around the arch. It takes practice, but the darker colour really emphasises the arch, widening the eyes.

## Top Treat
### Chanel Perfect Brows, £29
**Score: 8.43/10**
This complete grooming and make-up kit for brows has three shades of powder, for custom blending, along with a set of mini-tools: tweezers, brow brush, applicator plus a mirror.
**Comments:** 'Magnifying mirror means you catch the exact hair you want; fantastic tweezers – small but the tips are excellent' • 'colours are very good; you can vary the shades and depth for a natural daytime look, then stronger for evening' • 'you really can custom design the colour; the powder's easy to apply quite precisely' • 'lasted all day and evening'.

## Christian Dior Powder Eyebrow Pencil, £12
**Score: 8.3/10**
This powder-in-pencil-form has 'compacted' ingredients, delivering the naturalness of powder brow colour, with the ease and precision of a pencil – with a built-in grooming brush and a sharpener. In five shades, we tried 653 Blond.
**Comments:** 'Absolutely lovely: pencil soft and smooth, so very easy to make light feathery strokes; nice brush' • 'enhances brows rather than "making them up"; they look thicker and more even in colour' • 'liked the shimmery, natural-coloured powder' • 'loved this – could be applied lightly, or gave darker, more obvious line; stiff spiral brush really blended and shaped brows'.

# powders

## Shiseido Eyebrow and Eyeliner Compact, £19
**Score: 7.96/10**

Each compact has two shades of waxy powder, in three 'colour harmonies', and a double-ended applicator for 'soft but definite lines', according to Shiseido. Our testers used it as an eye-shadow, too – brilliant for a smoky effect, they say.

**Comments:** 'Smooth and even to apply, velvety feel, no dragging; nice compact with mirror, small applicator with thin ends so really easy to apply precisely; colours are natural, earthy shades'
• 'stubby brow brush was great for applying accurately' • 'sleek, sexy packaging; the black eyeliner made my hazel eyes look like sparkling emeralds!' • 'lovely soft consistency for brows; hint of waxiness made colour stick well'.

## *Beauty Steal* Clinique Eyebrow Pencil with Brush, £9
**Score: 7.88/10**

The closest to a 'Beauty Steal' we can find, this outranked any of the less expensive contenders by far. With a hard pencil formula, to avoid smudging or flaking, it also has a special brow-taming brush – though no sharpener – but is currently available only in dark brown.

**Comments:** 'Went on very easily and precisely; looked neutral and natural on – but gave definition'
• 'if I applied too heavily I gave brows a little brush to blend; looked really good' • 'lasted right

through a hot, sweaty, post-dancing night' • 'don't usually use a brow pencil, but this was easy, soft and gave a natural finish, and I use it all the time'.

## ✳ ✳ BareEscentuals BareMineral Essential Brow Kit, £26
**Score: 6.81**

Though quite a lot further down the charts, this powder version is the top choice in the brow category for anyone seeking a more natural brand of make-up. Available in four colours – our testers tried pale/ash blonde – and made from 100 per cent pure crushed minerals, it contains a brow colour, angled brow brush and a finishing gel, for grooming.

**Comments:** 'Very clear precise instructions: my heart sank when I saw the loose powder, but it was actually easy to apply' • 'stiff angled brush made application very easy if you tapped off excess before starting' • 'looked extremely natural; the more you use this, the easier it becomes; terrific' • 'gives a groomed, polished look'.

# eye make-up removers

A great eye make-up remover does all the work – with no rubbing and tugging, even if you're wearing waterproof mascara. One of the questions we're most frequently asked is, 'Which is the best remover?' So, while we have our own opinions (see below), here are our testers' completely independent reports

## WE LOVE...

Chanel Précision Eye Make-up Remover (right) has had a star role on Jo's bathroom shelf ever since it was launched: 'I've never found anything more efficient – the gorgeous packaging is just a bonus.' Sarah's supersensitive peepers have been known to revolt for days against removers, so she sticks to Prescriptives Quick Remover (our Top Treat) and Lancôme Bi-Facil Non Greasy Instant Cleanser for Sensitive Eyes, £16/125ml.

### Top Treat
### Prescriptives Quick Remover for Eye Makeup, £14/125ml

**Score: 9.16/10**

Not a single one of our testers reported any adverse reaction to this liquid formula, which is oil- and fragrance-free and infused with soothing cucumber extracts.

**Comments:** 'Wonderful – didn't need to rub at my eyes, which felt clean and fresh and ready for everything' • 'very refreshing: felt as if it had just been in the fridge – though it hadn't' • 'quickly removed all traces of eye make-up, skin felt smooth and conditioned' • 'great product – especially for people with sensitive eyes, like me'.

### Chanel Précision Eye Make-Up Remover, £13.50/100ml

**Score: 8.9/10**

This is a shake-vigorously-before-use product, rich in rose and cornflower waters – and comes in that oh-so-covetable Chanel packaging. It's Jo's absolute fave-rave remover, and has been for – oh, almost for ever.

**Comments:** 'This is an excellent product: it cleaned off eye make-up with no soreness and left skin moist: it didn't make my eyes water, unlike most eye make-up removers' • 'this felt luxurious and worked well – it didn't affect my contact lenses, either, which is a bonus' • 'removed make-up very easily – even two coats of mascara' • 'excellent: left the eye zone very moisturised after use – as if I'd used an eye cream: a real delight'.

## Sisley Gentle Make-Up Remover for Eyes & Lips, £25/125ml
**Score: 8.7/10**

Sisley, a luxury brand with a cult following, incorporate extracts of wild daisy, cornflower and soothing gardenia in this remover, and our testers particularly loved the straight-from-nature orange-blossom scent.

**Comments:** 'This one was a dream to use – no rubbing was needed, and all the gunk simply floated away – wonderful, magical stuff' • 'has a beautiful smell and refreshing on the eyes' • 'removed all traces of eye make-up very well, with slightly more effort on waterproof mascara' • 'very economical'.

## Simple Conditioning Eye Make Up Remover, £4.99/125ml
**Score: 7/10**

*Beauty Steal*

The no-nonsense Simple range is 100 per cent colour- and fragrance-free, and – in this case – the product is 100 per cent oil-free, too. The highest-scoring of the budget removers tested, it's formulated with kind-to-skin glycerine and Pro-Vitamin B5.

**Comments:** 'Very natural-seeming and simple – nothing to irritate the eyes' • 'I wear quite a bit of mascara, so I was impressed with how well this coped' • 'was calming on the delicate eye area and removed my eye make-up fairly effortlessly' • 'worked on lipstick, too'.

**tip** If you're decanting your eye make-up remover into a small bottle for travelling, shake it first: many removers today are what's called 'dual-phase' – meaning the oil and water blend only when shaken. If you don't do this, you'll end up with just the oil in your travel bottle, which can travel into your eyes, leaving them smeary.

## Jurlique OPC Make-up Remover, £23.25/100ml
**Score: 6.83/10**

The highest-scoring of the natural products we tested is actually intended as an all-over make-up remover milk, but our testers tried it specifically for one of its purposes: the removal of eye make-up. One of the founders of this all-natural Australian skincare brand used to work with Dr Hauschka, and these products contain herbs which have been grown on Jurlique's farm. In this remover, you'll find among the ingredients rosewood and lavender, plus antioxidant green tea, red wine grape seeds, vitamin E and turmeric.

**Comments:** 'No rubbing was required with this product, even for waterproof mascara – and it has a fantastic smell' • ' after use my skin felt moisturised and plump, soft and rehydrated' • 'I really loved the lavender/herbal scent of this one' • 'rich, creamy texture – the smell was fantastic and the skin round my eyes felt very smooth after I'd used this'.

# tweezers

Ooh, how you love a good pluck! Whoever would have thought that tweezers would score so highly among our testers? But certainly, all make-up artists agree: groomed brows widen the eyes and can give a 'mini-brow-lift' – and these ones make the job simple

Tweezers are highly individual: many of us start with the slanted version, and then 'graduate' to pointed tweezers once we're 'experts' – so there are winners of both types listed here. Though we tried some cheaper tweezers, none of those that scored well is particularly inexpensive. We'd say good tweezers are worth investing in – and worth keeping in a safe place, as they get damaged easily.

*Top Treat*

### Space NK Slant Tweezers, £15
**Score: 9.33/10**
From the own-label range by Space NK and available exclusively through their beautiques, mail order and website, these exceptionally high-scoring tweezers are individually crafted, with slanted ends which, Space NK say, 'permit an ideal positioning angle of the tweezers to the skin'. Several testers gave them full marks.
**Comments:** 'These are very easy to hold and comfortable to use: they don't move or slip in my hand' • 'quite fine blades, so you can select the exact hair you want to pluck; they work on even the really fine hairs other tweezers can't pick up' • 'I feel so confident with them that I've been practising on my friends' • 'I don't have to get my brows waxed any more' • 'the slant means it's easy to get a grip on individual hairs' • 'nice and sharp – a good point, and the tips actually met; liked the little wallet they come in'.

*tip* Our favourite make-up artists used to say aircraft loos had the best light for brow-plucking, but now tweezers are considered a potentially dangerous weapon – always pack in your suitcase, not hand luggage – so try your driving mirror instead. When you're stationary, of course.

## Tweezerman Slant Tip, £16

**Score: 9/10**

Tweezerman's tweezers, as used by celebs, make-up pros and beauty therapists, come with a useful lifetime guarantee, so when they begin to feel blunt they can be sent off, re-sharpened and returned – an idea we truly applaud. Available with several shapes and grips, including a wide-grip, the slant tip wowed our pluckers.

**Comments:** 'The sort of tweezers that become firm friends! They make all kinds of facial hair extraction easy and addictive!' • 'surprised at how easy and precise these tweezers were; could remove much shorter regrowth than with pointed ones' • 'blown away with these beauties: they move at the perfect angle which protects you from the sharp edges; the root comes too, so less plucking and longer results' • 'like the rubber cap and plastic holder, great for carrying around'.

## Shavata Precision Tweezers, £19.50

**Score: 8.1/10**

Created and used by one of Britain's 'brow gurus', Shavata, this is a point-tipped tweezer manufactured in Switzerland by a factory that makes tools for producing precision watches.

**Comments:** 'Quite simply the best tweezers I've ever used' • 'very sleek, cool, professional; fiddly at first, but when you get used to them much more precise' • 'sharp and fine enough to make plucking fine re-growth a breeze' • 'I felt completely groomed' • 'very impressed at how pain free the tweezers made plucking'.

## *Beauty Steal* Ruby & Millie Narrow Slanted Tweezers, £10.50

**Score: 8.1/10**

These are the closest thing you will find to a 'Beauty Steal' in this category: hand-finished, slanted tweezers – 'narrow but not pointy' said

one tester – made for this make-up artist duo by Tweezerman, which come with a safety cap and useful resealable wallet.

**Comments:** 'Excellent grip, and the angled tip makes it easy to get the chosen hair' • 'took out those invisible hairs which spoil the look of your eye shadow' • 'tweezer tips meet accurately, so the hairs are caught firmly, with minimal pressure' • 'like the stylish matt steel grey finish'.

## Estée Lauder Artist's Brow Stylist Mobile Essentials Kit, £18

**Score: 7.71**

Our panellists liked the mini-tweezers that came with this nifty, portable kit from Lauder, which also includes a brow brush, dual-ended brow pencil and tube of brow gel, and is available in shades of light or medium brown.

**Comments:** ' I just loved the kit; having tweezers and brow brush in one compact is great' • 'loved the mini-tweezers – a bit fiddly, but they're easy to carry in your handbag to keep brows groomed' • 'dinky innovative packaging; tweezers were good for touching up odd stray hairs'.

# eyelash curlers

For us, you can file eyelash curlers under 'life's too short', except for special occasions, but we know plenty of women who absolutely swear by them. Many of the panellists who trialled these were 'eyelash curler virgins' – but were highly impressed. Most of the high scorers were 'manual' curlers, but we've included a review of the top 'heated' lash-curler, as these are increasingly popular

**WE LOVE…**

When Jo does opt for lash-curling – 'it hardly seems worth it, as mine are so sparse!' – she's a fan of the Model Co Lash Wand (opposite), which she finds delivers a great curl. And Sarah – well, she just isn't evolved enough to use them.

**Top Treat**
### Shu Uemura Eyelash Curlers, £16
**Score: 8.3/10**

Can't say we were surprised that these curlers romped home first; they've earned a place in the Beauty Hall of Fame, and are rightly described by Shu Uemura as 'the Rolls-Royce of make-up artist accessories'. The soft, durable rubber eliminates any risk of lash-breakage, and makes for maximum curl with minimum effort.

**Comments:** 'Lashes looked longer and more dramatic – I'm definitely a convert' • 'very easy to use and comfortable to hold' • 'with mascara, my short lashes looked really full' • 'lashes were double length and really curly – an absolutely amazing product, brilliant!'

**Beauty Steal**
### Tweezerman Classic Eyelash Curler, £7
**Score: 7.88/10**

Like Shu Uemura, Tweezerman have an incredibly high reputation for their make-up accessories, which are often quoted as 'celebrity must-haves'. Tweezerman offer replacement rubber tips for these curlers, which (like the Shu Uemura design) have a 'scissor' grip.

**Comments:** 'Very easy instructions; took a maximum of ten seconds to curl my lashes, a huge improvement on my others' • 'gave a soft natural curl, not a "crimped" look' • 'made my eyes look more wide awake and slightly brighter' • 'these are amazing and don't even need heating; they seem more expensive than other metal curlers because there is a soft cushioned feel when you squeeze the handles together'.

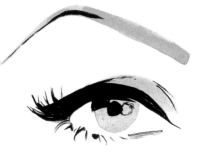

## *Beauty Steal* Mister Mascara Wide Eye Lash Curler, £7.50
### Score: 7/10

The clever thing about these lash curlers is the fact that they're made of transparent plastic, which – especially for novices – makes it easier to see what you're doing. Helpfully, there is a refill rubber pad integrated into the handle, for whenever it needs replacing.

**Comments:** 'This was absolutely fabulous: application was comfortable and easy, and the effects were gorgeous' • 'mascara was easier to apply, my lashes were more defined and my eyes looked wider – I was impressed' • 'this was the first time I've ever used one, but I'd definitely give it room in my make-up bag now' • 'the curl lasted for well over 12 hours and lots of people said how great my eyes looked'.

## Model Co Lash Wand, £25
### Score: 7/10

The best of the battery-operated heated curlers, this is a sleek silver cylinder with a mascara-like wand on the end – and it's become a favourite with beauty editors. Most lash curlers work by 'clamping' the lashes, but with the heated kind, you switch them on, wait for them to warm up, then 'stroke' through the lashes – just like mascara. The thought may be a bit scary, but they don't get so hot as to burn the skin.

**Comments:** 'Nothing short of absolutely fabulous' • 'with mascara as well, my eyes looked fabulous and lots of people commented' • 'curl lasted nearly two days even after showering' • 'eyelashes looked very long and luscious – certainly the most effective and easiest-to-use lash curler that I have ever come across' • 'boyfriend comment on my "flicky" eyelashes, so it must have been really noticeable!'

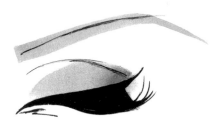

# lip glosses

Like most women, we're totally addicted to lip glosses – they cheer us up almost as much as a new pair of shoes –  and are a lot easier on the bank balance! Finding the perfect gloss – not too sticky, and which won't wear off before you've taken your first sip of cappuccino – is a challenge, though. Our testers slicked their way through more than 50 glosses to come up with the following verdicts

**WE LOVE…**

Jo is a fan of Aveda Lip Shine; she is also a recent convert to Clinique Colour Surge Impossibly Glossy, £11/14ml. Sarah always loves DiorKiss, £14/10ml, in Praline. And of course, we're both sold on our own Beauty Bible Pink Lip Gloss by Prescriptives, £20, from Harrods.

*Top Treat*

## Yves Saint Laurent Lisse Gloss, £14.50
**Score: 8.9/10**

An exceptionally high score for this stylishly packaged winner, which comes in a choice of four shades, designed to moisturise as well as gloss. The secret nourishing ingredient, according to YSL, is 'Gold of Pleasure' oil, from the camelina plant.
**Comments:** 'Loved the texture – really smooth' • 'gave lips a full, fresh look' • 'very creamy and not at all sticky' • 'a firm wand with a good shape that gives you lots of control' • 'nice "click" to the packaging' • 'made lips look full and kissable!'

## Guerlain Divinora Kiss Kiss Gloss, £14
**Score: 8.61/10**

The sheer elegance of the packaging, which has a 'beaten' gold lid, and the ultra-moisturising comfy-to-wear texture earned this rave reviews.
**Comments:** 'The glamour puss of lip glosses! I felt proud to have it in my make-up bag' • 'great applicator – easy to apply without mirror' • 'I started out thinking this was over-priced – but the more I used it, the more I liked it' • 'loved this gloss – very glam and lasted well' • 'lips felt nourished'.

## Molton Brown Wonderlips Gloss, £19
**Score: 8.05/10**

Molton Brown have incorporated their 'Maxi-lip™' patented technology into this gloss, which is claimed to 'boost lip definition' – but our panel of testers was generally more impressed by the long-lasting shine than its 'volumising' action. It comes in six shades.

**Comments:** 'I loved this – great texture, great sheen' • 'looks, feels and tastes natural – perfect' • 'gave fab coverage and looked good through the day' • 'lovely velvety consistency'.

## Paul & Joe, £14
### Score: 8.05/10

The gorgeous flower-embossed tube whispers 'boudoir beauty'. From the make-up range by Parisian designers Paul & Joe, it comes in 12 pout-worthy shades.

**Comments:** 'Very easy to apply, with a good brush – the handle is etched, giving a good grip' • 'amazingly moisturising – lips feel soft, supple and nourished for at least an hour after gloss wore off completely' • 'glorious packaging' • 'divine smell – a bit like strawberry shortcake!' • 'really good coverage with just one coat'.

 ## Revlon Super Lustrous® Lip Gloss, £6.49
### Score: 7.27/10

Contains 'LiquiSilk™', a special blend of aloe and vitamins for silky-smooth lips, with an angled sponge-tip wand.

**Comments:** 'Very pretty, party-ish gloss' • 'very comfortable – just the right consistency' • 'my thin lips looked a little fuller' • 'extremely glamorous' • 'lips feel lovely and smooth' • 'I really loved the packaging – very Agent Provocateur'.

 ## Rimmel Jelly Gloss, £3.49
### Score: 7.27/10

'High-shine, wet-look and non-sticky' are Rimmel's claims for this very affordably priced, fruity-flavoured gloss, which is available in five shades plus a clear version, and which

 **tip** Gloss wears off notoriously fast – but Jeanine Lobel, founder of Stila, has this tip: 'Line lips with a co-ordinating lip liner first, then "fill in" by drawing all over the lip with the liner. The liner will make the lips matt and provide a base for the gloss, so it doesn't slip and slide so much.'

tied with Revlon's gloss as the joint 'Beauty Steal' in this category.

**Comments:** 'A lovely berry taste, and very comfortable to wear' • 'comfortable without being tacky – makes the lips feel really soft' • 'very sheer and pretty' • 'a great girly product with a fun fruit flavour' • 'such nice packaging – just like Juicy Tubes!'.

## Aveda Lip Shine, £11.50
### Score: 7.05/10

The most natural of our winners, this wet-look gloss is packed with nourishing fruit and vegetable extracts (including beetroot), together with an organic 'berry lipid' moisture complex based on vitamin E, cranberry, bilberry and blueberry. In a choice of seven shades, it delivers a breath-freshening zing of peppermint, cinnamon, anise and basil, too. A big favourite of Jo's for its naturalness.

**Comments:** 'Very good moisturising effect – in fact, I'd use this instead of lip balm' • 'the only gloss out of the ones that I tested which didn't make my lips tingle or sting at all' • 'lovely sheer colour' • 'this one lasted right the way through a Big Mac meal!' • 'if I'm going to end up eating lip gloss along with my food, I'd rather it be natural than all-petroleum jelly!'

# lip balms

Fact: chapped lips just aren't gorgeous – let alone comfortable. Since it's easy to spend a small fortune 'auditioning' to find the best lip balm, our testers have done the legwork – or lipwork – for you, and have declared these pout protectors to be the best

L ips are one of the most exposed, yet most delicate areas of skin, with a very thin outer layer and few sebaceous glands, making them ultra-vulnerable to wind, cold, sun and central heating. We like to tuck a lip balm in every pocket and bag for outdoors – with an extra pot on our desks and bedside tables. If you're concerned about the fact that you basically 'eat' lip balm, you might want to check the list of ingredients and consider the natural 'daisied' options below.

## WE LOVE…

Jo is mostly faithful to all-natural **Dr Hauschka Lip Care Stick, £7**, and **Intensive Lip Treatment**, from a small New Zealand natural beauty company called **Trilogy, £6.95**. Additionally, Sarah likes **Liz Earle's Superbalm** (see page 81) and **Aveda's Lip Saver** (right).

*Top Treat*

## ❋ Aveda Lip Saver ™ SPF15, £7
Score: 8.5/10

Aveda's high-scoring entry relies on beeswax and other natural waxes to seal in moisture. It's a waterproof formula, in a twist-up stick, with a refreshing twist of cinnamon leaf, clove and anise oils, offering the bonus of an SPF15 sunscreen and antioxidants to shield vulnerable skin.

**Comments:** 'Loved the honey taste and smell – my lips felt wonderful, very moisturised and hydrated' • 'dramatic moisturisation: didn't need to reapply for 24 hours' • 'lips felt plumper and fuller, especially if dabbed on at night' • 'lipstick lasts longer with this as a base' • 'liked the clear formulation with waxy protective texture'.

## Crème de la Mer Lip Balm, £35/9g

**Score: 8.31/10**

Probably the world's most luxuriously priced lip balm, but our testers loved it. From the 'cult' Crème de la Mer skincare range, it features a high concentration of the special marine algae 'broth' in the skin cream itself, plus a lipid complex, to moisturise, and a jolt of mint, to soothe discomfort.
**Comments:** 'terrific! Loved the vanilla/mint scent; one application kept lips moisturised all day' • 'elegant packaging, perfect texture' • 'can use over lipstick, too, to set colour and moisturise' • 'pure luxury! I wanted to keep on applying it; plumped lips slightly; left them very soft, with a nice gleam' • 'lips softer and smoother over a week'.

## Prescriptives Lip Specialist, £12

**Score: 8.22/10**

This teensy pot of high-powered action contains naturally derived oils – macadamia, avocado, olive, and apricot plus shea butter – but petrochemicals, as well. If it is used longer term, Prescriptives say, it will help diminish fine lines *along* the lip line.
**Comments:** 'Can I give it 11 out of 10? Made my usually dry lips feel yummy' • 'gave my lips a nice sheen' • 'my boyfriend kept stealing this!' • 'really does soothe and smooth' • 'after a month, my lips are much softer and smoother'.

 **Barbara Daly's Make-up for Tesco Luminous Lip Care, £5.50**

**Score: 7.9/10**

Clever! This is a balm and a gloss in one – created by make-up genius Barbara Daly for her signature range – which conditions lips while the pink, light-reflecting particles add a hint of a tint, creating the illusion of a 'plumped-up' pout.
**Comments:** 'Lovely soft pink shimmer, so can be worn on its own; also looked really pretty over

 **tip** If chapped lips are a problem, apply balm before sleep, so the emollient ingredients can work their magic while you're not constantly licking your lips. Also, if you have a cold, try smearing lip balm round your nose to stop that post-sniffle cracking and flaking. Not very glamorous, but effective.

a lipstick' • 'moisturised well and lips felt plumper and in good condition' • 'good protection in the sun; easy to apply, very light, but stops cracking' • 'pretty packaging, quite expensive looking; balm a lot less sticky than most – and lasts longer than gloss' • 'as good as a lipstick: your lips look made up, but in a very subtle, natural way'.

 **Neal's Yard Organic Herbal Lip Balm, £2.50**

**Score: 7.87/10**

If you want something that's literally good enough to eat on your lips – and we certainly do – you'll want to know about the highest-scoring of the certified organic products that our testers tried. This little pot offers soothing and healing calendula, comfrey and lavender with skin-toning lemon and myrrh, in a protective and vitamin-rich soya oil, wheatgerm, sunflower and beeswax base.
**Comments:** 'Can't fault this: my lips are definitely in better condition – lovely citrus aroma, and a good base for lipstick' • 'my builder son and his mates say it's brilliant for their chapped lips' • 'I'm going to throw out all my other lip balms and only use this nourishing product' • 'as always, Neal's Yard produce quality for a very reasonable price'.

# lip liners

Think lip liner and you might think 'ghastly aubergine lines around pale lips'. But in the right shade – as close to your natural lip colour as you can find it – a lip liner can enhance your lip shape, prevent 'bleeding' and help your lipstick or gloss stay put

**WE LOVE…**

When Jo tried Clinique Sheer Shaper, £11, her reaction was: 'Why didn't anyone think of this before?' It's transparent, so it gives a more subtle line, and is great under lip gloss: now she won't use anything else. Sarah loves lip liners too, especially good for – ahem! – more mature lips. Her fave is Pixi Lip Define Duo No 1, £11, a slim pencil, natural pinky brown at one end and a deeper tone – for evenings, maybe – at the other.

Where most women go wrong is to match their lip liner to their lipstick, rather than to their natural lip tone: with the latter, when your lipstick wears off, there's no obvious outline. So we made sure that our panels – each of ten testers – trialled neutral, suits-all-skintones shades. Of the dozens of lip pencils our different panels tried, these performed best.

Several winning products were more chunky crayon than trad pencils. A few testers commented that these give a not-so-precise line, but lots raved about them as an all-over-the-mouth base, which made lippie (applied on top) last much longer – four or five times, said one tester – and also looked great with a clear lip gloss.

**Top Treat**

## NARS Lipliner Pencil, £13
### Score: 8.22/10

François Nars is a renowned make-up artist whose signature make-up line comes in very stylish packaging. He clearly disagrees with our advice about matching lip liner to lip colour rather than lipstick, because this crayon-sized pencil comes in 21 shades – we're not budging, though! Our testers tried the shade Bahama. **Comments:** 'A great product, versatile, easy to use, went on smoothly and evenly, and gave a soft natural outline' • 'I've never used a lip pencil before but was really impressed with this – gave my lips a much more professional look and continued making my lips appear good even when the top lipstick faded' • 'I used it as a base and it improved the texture of my lips' • 'waxy and velvety texture' • 'I really loved this, both as a lip liner and as a lipstick – either alone or with a shimmery gloss on top'.

**If you find lip liner or lipstick drying, always prep your lips with balm first and let it sink in for at least ten minutes.**

## ☀ ☀ BareEscentuals Lip Liner, £12
**Score: 7.7/10**

BareEscentuals is one of the few truly natural make-up lines on the market, based on crushed mineral pigments – along with waxes, where a product requires a soft texture, as with this lip pencil. Designed to be long-lasting, these creamy crayon lip liners are available only in what BareEscentuals describe as 'universally wearable, classic shades' – our testers' shade was Nude, which suited most of them.

**Comments:** 'This is a great product! It has a smooth creamy texture that glides on effortlessly. It can be very precise – or create a full pouty lip outline, if you prefer' • 'wonderful lip base: my lipstick lasted almost all day without reapplying and it's so creamy my lips felt moisturised' • 'nude colour goes with any shade – a real desert island must-have' • 'made neutral lipstick look much better – more noticeable and "finished"'.

### Beauty Steal — Miss Sporty Mini-Me Lip Liner, £2.29
**Score: 7.65/10**

A fantastic score for surely one of the greatest beauty bargains to be found anywhere on the planet: this product is absolutely teensy – with a price tag to match – yet brilliantly does the job of outlining lips, with its velvety-soft formulation. A bonus is that it doesn't need sharpening. In case you've never heard of them, Miss Sporty are part of Coty's beauty empire. The shade our testers tried was Toffee.

**Comments:** 'This was easy to apply, very smooth and even, easy to be precise' • 'it was great not to have to sharpen it' • 'I liked the softer-than-my-usual outline – less Joan Collins' • 'held on lip colour well: I couldn't lick it off as quickly as I can with most lipsticks' • 'worked really well as a base for lipstick' • 'easy to drop into a pocket or purse'.

## Clinique Cream Shaper for Lips, £11
**Score: 7.25/10**

The 'cream' in the name is just there to distinguish this fragrance-free, hypoallergenic product from another lip pencil that was launched at the same time, Clinique Sheer Shaper – which didn't score so well with our pouting panellists, but happens to be Jo's fave (see opposite). Cream Shaper comes with a small brush, too, which made it straightforward to use as a lip base.

**Comments:** 'I loved this – one of the best lip pencils I've ever used, not at all hard and goes on with no effort; needs sharpening often – but I'll be buying this for ever!' • 'very natural finish' • 'as a lipstick, with gloss on top, lasted from breakfast to lunch, at least four hours' • 'very easy to use, good sized "nib"' • 'incredibly easy to apply, precisely because it went on so smoothly so you could get a continuous line'.

# long-lasting lipsticks

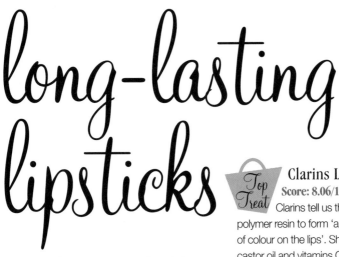

Hurrah: there are now lipsticks out there which survive meals, drinks, kissing – but don't leave your lips as dehydrated as if you'd stepped off a 24-hour flight or camel-trekked across the Sahara. But there's a but – or two. As 'stay-put-ability' is pretty high-tech and relies on synthetic ingredients, would-be natural beauties will have to put up with reapplying their usual (natural) wax-based lipstick, because none of those we tested could be awarded even a single 'daisy' for naturalness. There's no real 'Beauty Steal', either – though the Max Factor lippies come closest: we're paying for expensive technology in this category

*Top Treat*

## Clarins Le Rouge, £13.50
**Score: 8.06/10**
Clarins tell us this uses an innovative polymer resin to form 'a sheer, adherent microfilm of colour on the lips'. Shea butter, wheatgerm oil, castor oil and vitamins C and E nourish, soften and protect lips, while Clarins also claim their product's creamy texture and glossy shine will make lips look smoother, plumper and fuller. There are 38 shades, altogether.
**Comments:** 'Lips felt hydrated and wonderfully smooth – fabulous' • 'survived tea and a banana' • 'looks and feels fantastic' • 'left lips in lovely condition' • 'love the classy packaging – very eyecatching' • 'plumped lips, making them appear very full – and colour stays true'.

## Max Factor Lipfinity, £9.99
**Score: 7.6/10**
This innovative two-step process, designed to last up to eight hours, involves firstly 'painting on' intense colour with Permatone™ , a complex that 'attaches' colour (27 shades) to lips, with 'a flexible mesh effect', then sets in 60 seconds. Next, slick on the moisturising, dewy, balm-like top coat, which should be touched up during the day. However, most testers commented that, when used regularly, their lips became drier.
**Comments:** 'Ten out of ten – didn't budge after the first drink, and there was still colour left when

**Comments:** 'Stain dries extremely fast and is quite dry, but once you put the gloss on it is wonderful and moist' • 'lasted through three drinks and lunch' • 'no lipstick marks on cups: lasts for ages and the gloss is stunning, so moisturising' • 'lasted for 11 hours after the initial application!'

### Elizabeth Arden Exceptional Lipstick, £13.50
**Score: 7.2/10**

This creamy formulation apparently takes the technology for its long-lastingness from the ink industry, combining that staying power with the nourishing effect of moisturising ceramides, which are a bit of an Arden signature. There are 24 shades to choose from.

**Comments:** 'Exceptional indeed – long lasting, with a fabulous colour, and moisturising, too' • 'altogether, it lasted two tea breaks and through to after lunch' • 'a beautiful, lasting finish' • 'moisturised and looked stunning'.

### Shiseido The Makeup Staying Power Moisturising Lipstick, £15
**Score: 7.15/10**

Shiseido claim that this features ten times more glycerine than regular moisturising lipsticks, to keep colour glossy and vibrant hour-after-hour. It makes it more comfortable, too. In a choice of eight shades, it boasts a combination of 'staying polymers, moisturising capsules and lasting oil'.

**Comments:** 'A just-kissed look emerges as this fades – I liked it a lot' • 'lots of compliments when I wore this' • 'amazing – not a single trace on my cup after two drinks' • 'lustrous, moisture-rich finish' • 'excellent staying power without looking too heavy' • 'nice packaging, so convenient to apply'.

I went to bed' • 'today I reapplied moisture stick three times in the morning, cleaned teeth, drank about three coffees, had lunch and it's still looking good' • 'colour was very good and faded nicely'.

### Max Factor Lipfinity Everlites, £9.99
**Score: 7.3/10**

The new 'baby sister' to the original Lipfinity (see opposite), this is the most lightweight formulation yet for a long-last lipstick, designed to last up to a stunning ten hours. It works in the same two-stage way as the original, but is sheerer, with a lighter-weight feel. The topcoat includes 'Glossamer', a shine-boosting ingredient that gives a soft feel and glossy look and is designed to be reapplied during the day. In 15 shades.

# lip-plumpers

Women dream of a miracle product that will give them superkissable Angelina Jolie lips. Well, nothing but collagen injections will do that – and, frankly, we wouldn't go there – but, according to our panellists, these lip-plumpers really do have a pout-enhancing effect

WE LOVE...

Jo doesn't bother with a lip-plumper but swears by Guerlain Divinora Lip Pencil in Cupidon, £12, a lightly pearlised pale pink pencil, which she uses to outline her cupid's bow. And Sarah can report that Prescriptives Beauty Bible Pink Treatment Lip Gloss, £20, does the kissable trick quite perfectly, with a touch of Touche Eclat or Dior SkinFlash in the top 'V' for special effects.

We lumped together different types of product here: lip 'cosmetics' with light-reflective pigments and waxes, some with warming ingredients that 'puff up' lips, and others claiming to stimulate the production of collagen. None scored really highly but our testers were mostly impressed enough to say they'd buy these again.

*Top Treat*

## Lancôme Primordiale Optimum Lèvres, £21.50
Score: 7.79/10

After a single application, Lancôme promise, 'lips feel softer, better hydrated and easier to make up.' And lipstick should last longer, too, they add. Key ingredients in this anti-ageing treatment are pure vitamin E, a red seaweed extract, and 'Flexium' (based on nourishing waxes, oils and powders). **Comments:** 'My lipstick almost glided on; no feathering or bleeding – and stayed in place longer than normal; fantastic!' • 'definitely made the lip outline stand out more – lips fuller – very Liz Hurley!' • 'lips rehydrated – and look younger' • 'gave extra definition to the outline of my mouth'.

## Estée Lauder FX Lip Amplifying Base, £12.50
Score: 7.66/10

From Lauder's new range of primers – designed to help us mere mortals create professional make-up results – comes this: a liquid, based on micro-sponge technology, with wand applicator, which smooths away fine lines and, say Lauder, makes lips appear more voluminous, while also priming them to lock in colour. Plus, there's an antioxidant blend to help protect against environmental damage. Testers were surprised by the significant volumising effect.

**Comments:** 'My lips were genuinely fuller'; • 'gave my lips a naturally plumper look, starting after about 30 seconds; helped to fix lipstick longer than normal' • 'I really liked this product: my lips were plumped up and had more natural colour to them; the little lines on your lips were "pushed out" to make lips smoother and bigger – the effect was especially noticeable on my top lip' • 'this is the business – gives you that model finish'.

### L'Oréal Paris Glam' Shine, £6.99
**Score: 7.6/10**

This non-sticky gloss is described by L'Oréal Paris as a sparkling, semi-transparent lip colour, with a visible lip-plumping effect. With a fruity fragrance, it comes in a wide range of shades, including 'Crystal', which changes colour depending on the angle you view it from.

**Comments:** 'My lips looked shiny, fuller, softer – and very kissable!' • 'glamorous and shining, sparkly and special' • 'lovely and moist' • 'overall, this was an excellent product'.

## Molton Brown Wonder Lips Gloss, £19
**Score: 7.15/10**

Molton Brown issue limited-edition seasonal shades of this gloss alongside a selection of classic shades. A mirror-shine gloss, they tell us it's 'enriched with Maxi-lip™ technology, to boost lip definition, condition and 'up to 40 per cent

**tip** Anyone with thin lips can use lip liner – very carefully – to extend the outline of their lips, make-up pro Vincent Longo once told us. The secret is to draw just along the outer edge of the lip line and always to finish the line exactly in the corner of the lips – that way you avoid the Ronald McDonald effect.

moisture-volume', when used over time. There's shea butter in there, too.

**Comments:** 'Loved this – I have quite full lips and it made them look even plumper' • 'lips looked very full, glossy, smooth and kissable' • 'I loved this – husband said my lips looked very kissable!' • 'nice gloss, not too sticky, comfortable on lips'.

## Philosophy Big Mouth, £16
**Score: 7.05**

The tingling effect of this gloss, from Philosophy's 'Unplastic Surgery' range, comes from menthol, which creates a feeling and look, albeit temporary – the time varied with individuals – of fullness. The formula features topical vitamins to help soften and smooth, and comes in two shades, 'Pink' and 'Nude' – which our testers were assigned – to be worn alone or under a favourite lip colour.

**Comments:** 'My mother couldn't believe it and said my lips looked *totally* fuller. No collagen needed!' • 'very comfortable, and I got a lot of compliments from friends while wearing this' • 'tasted slightly mentholy, fruity – nice' • 'gloss gives a great natural colour boost, making lips very kissable – and subtly plumps them, too'.

# pressed powders

If your face tends to glow, pressed powder is a beauty essential for on-the-go touch-ups. (Drier complexions may not need it.) In search of the perfect pressed powder, our teams of ten testers tried literally dozens of compacts, of which the ones on these pages were the (anti-)shining examples

## WE LOVE...

Jo prefers the cream-to-powder effect of her favourite compact foundation (see page 29); powders always look dusty on her ultra-dry skin. Sarah hasn't used them for years – but may have to try again in view of the favourable comments.

W here companies offer a translucent shade, which should work on every skin from Nordic pale to black, we asked to test those. Where a spectrum of shades is available, we requested ten of the palest hue and sent them to appropriate panels. Many testers said they preferred applying powder with a brush initially, then a sponge or pad while out and about.

 Top Treat

## Stila Sheer Color Face Powder SPF15, £18

Score: 8.05/10

In a chic silver compact, make-up artist Jeanine Lobel's creation 'is the answer to oily skin's prayers', she tells us, helping to shield skin from UV rays while blotting shine (it has an SPF15). Our testers trialled the Shade 1 (of two) option, formulated for fair-to-medium skintones.

**Comments:** 'Excellent: covers shiny bits well and you can easily reapply without it looking cakey. Like the SPF15' • 'lovely silky-feel face powder – gave a finished look to make-up and kept shine at bay longer than my usual product' • 'looked incredibly pale but gave a very natural finish' • 'helped balance my skin tone and set my foundation' • 'absorbed excess oil without looking too powdery'.

## Clinique Gentle Light Pressed Powder, £20

**Score: 7.97/10**

This is the pressed version of the loose powder that came out top in that category (see overleaf), – no mean feat for one product to do so well for both formulations. Silicones give it a weightless, silky feel, there's vitamin E to help guard against environmental damage – and a 'jet-milled process' ensures the teensiest particle size of the mica and talc. It also features Clinique's 'Gentle Reflection Technology', said to give a line-blurring, softening result. In five shades.

**Comments:** 'Fantastic! I've never used any powder over make-up before and am very impressed; no dryness whatsoever and my skin felt super soft and silky and definitely looked more even' • 'definitely a must for all make-up bags' • 'ideal for day or night wear, very versatile' • 'my face didn't look floury at all' • 'I love it!'

 **Dr Hauschka Face Powder Finale Compact, £18**

**Score: 7.83/10**

A very high score for this powder, which features a high content of silk (alongside talc and mica) for a matt finish. Lightly rose fragranced and said to be fine for even the touchiest skins, it comes in one, universal (Translucent) shade.

**Comments:** 'Fabulously fine, divine-smelling powder that gives a lovely softness to my skin • 'great finish, natural, totally matt, evened skin tone' • 'gave my combination skin a long-lasting finish' • 'set my make-up to perfection'.

## Bobbi Brown Sheer Finish Face Powder, £22

**Score: 7.75/10**

Our friend Bobbi Brown pioneered the idea of 'yellow pigments' in face powder, which are said

to be more flattering to most skintones than pink pigments. The mattifying effect comes from cornstarch, and our testers tried the Pale Yellow shade (from a range of six), a real beauty classic.

**Comments:** 'Really lovely product, perfect "nude" colour, incredibly sheer, as perfect for a no-make-up look as it was for the full works, very long lasting' • 'I don't usually use powder but will use this because you can't see it and my make-up lasts longer' • 'stylish, expensive-looking packaging' • 'loved this; good at setting make-up and worked well to mattify nose and forehead'.

 **L'Oréal Translucide Compact Powder, £7.99**

**Score: 6.75/10**

The highest-scoring of the budget pressed powders, this came in some way down, but we've included it because we know it's not always possible to splurge on pricier brands. It comes with a mirror and soft sponge applicator, and the formula has 'micro-fine light reflecting powders to give a radiant glow', say L'Oréal.

**Comments:** 'Lovely lightweight powder that gives a natural translucent matt finish with a sheen' • 'leaves skin silky and set my make-up; kept cream blusher in place all day' • 'worked well on shiny zones' • 'natural finish and balanced skin tone' • 'really nice silky powder; didn't cover up my broken thread veins, but did work on a few blotchy patches'.

*tip* If your powder comes with a pouch, use it, don't lose it! It helps 'buffer' the contents from cracking when you drop your make-up bag/handbag.

65

# loose powders

Powdering your face may sound old fashioned, but make-up artists today still recommend loose powder for setting foundation, both for day and evening. It isn't practical for on-the-go touch-ups, though, so we've also tested pressed powders – see pages 64-5

T he new light-as-a-feather loose powders are virtually undetectable and shouldn't cake or clog pores. Apply with a velvet sponge or with a brush, which tends to give a lighter finish, in our experience. To prevent your powder brush picking up too much powder, don't dip it into the powder itself – just swoop it around the inside of the lid. Some brands offer powder shades that are matched to foundations – but we'd recommend choosing a translucent product as a one-shade-suits-all choice, especially if you're not used to wearing powder. Even our testers with dark and Asian skins were pleasantly surprised to find that the translucent ones they tried worked well for them.

**Top Treat**

## Clinique Gentle Light Powder, £18.50
Score: 8.2/10

This has a unique 'gentle reflection technology', based on mosaic-like mirrored particles, to make skins appear luminous while minimising flaws like redness and discoloration. It comes in five shades, all hypo-allergenic and fragrance-free.
**Comments:** 'Honestly, this enhanced my complexion 150 per cent – gave a wonderful glow and lasted five hours before a re-touch was needed' • 'excellent, natural finish – it even seemed to minimise the appearance of pores' • 'this made my skin look younger, softer and less lined' • 'make-up didn't look white or chalky, and foundation better than ever before'.

## Lancôme Poudre Majeur Excellence, £21.50
Score: 7.7/10

Poudre Majeur Excellence, in six shades, is the updated version of Lancôme's bestselling Poudre Majeur, with the same light-capturing powers, for a face-illuminating satin-smooth finish.
**Comments:** 'Usually my make-up rubs off by lunchtime but it stayed on all day' • 'fine and silky texture – I'm often put off by the way powders look like ground-up chalk' • 'my face looked very natural – no unevenness, and it didn't settle into lines' • 'I don't usually use face powder, but this one has converted me'.

## Becca Fine Loose Finishing Powder, £28

**Score: 7.5/10**

This Australian make-up artist's brand created by Rebecca Morrice-Williams offers a huge choice of shades to match every skin tone. Our panellists tested one of the lightest shades, packaged in Becca's stylish mocha.

**Comments:** 'Looked like I'd had a professional artist do my make-up' • 'beautifully silky texture' • 'the matt effect lasted a long time' • 'lovely natural finish delivered a balanced skin tone' • 'very impressive – since trying this powder I've bought other Becca products'.

## Chanel Natural Finish Loose Powder, £22.50

**Score: 7.47/10**

Chanel promise this sheer, matt powder will deliver 'outstanding glide and comfort during application'. It comes in the usual gorgeous Chanel packaging, complete with velvet puff and a small sieve to prevent spillage.

**Comments:** 'Covered up blemishes, balanced skin tone, made my face look flawless' • 'really nice texture – velvety doesn't come close; loved the radiant effect' • 'very natural looking, with a lustre' • 'I'll buy this if I have to remortgage!'

## Stila Loose Powder, £18

**Score: 7.1/10**

From make-up pro Jeanine Lobel's range, this loose powder comes in a small aluminium canister with a twist top like a talc shaker, which makes it spill-proof for carrying in a handbag.

**Comments:** 'I was very impressed with the shine control' • 'this "set" my make-up – but in a very natural way, and it lasted longer than usual' • 'my skin looked silky all over with this' • 'I found it just perfect for daytime touch-ups'.

## T LeClerc Poudre Libre, £26

**Score: 7.1/10**

This cult powder dates back to 1881 and the metal boxes are still filled by hand. From the 22 shades that are available, we sent our testers 'Banane' – a soft, very pale yellow that claims to soften and brighten a tired face.

**Comments:** 'My make-up lasted all day – which it never does, normally; people kept asking me if I'd re-done it' • 'great finish, and my skin looked natural – and the packaging is really pretty, too' • 'luxurious packaging, wonderful coverage – and it managed to keep my shine at bay'.

##  Corn Silk Original Satin Face Powder, £6.75

**Score: 7.1/10**

A make-up pros' favourite – and a real beauty classic – Corn Silk gets its mattifying effect from powdered walnut shells.

**Comments:** 'Helped to balance skin tone, even when not wearing foundation' • 'silky smooth – a brilliant find; I was really impressed' • 'very natural finish with a tiny sparkle – very pretty' • 'the black and gold packaging make you feel as though you've raided your mother's make-up bag'.

## Aveda Loose Powder, £15

**Score: 6.35/10**

This fragrant talc-free product in just two shades contains powdered minerals to illuminate, plus skin-nourishing resveratrol from grapes. Although it didn't score highly with all our testers, the ones who loved it – well, they loved it.

**Comments:** 'Cut shine on my oily T-zone very well' • 'a good natural finish with a little sheen that left my skin glow-y' • 'gave a nice finished look to make-up for the evening' • 'the inner lid with holes controls how much you get, and stops powder going everywhere' • 'beautiful rose aroma'.

# facial mists

These do triple duty: cooling us down on a hot day – or long flight – and 'setting' or 'refreshing' make-up. The perfect facial mist is like English mizzle, leaving skin dewy and plump. But a badly designed one makes you look like you've just been in a downpour (result: runny mascara). How to choose? Just read on…

We'd personally categorise these as beauty non-essentials – though we like them for stuffy offices, heat waves or travelling – but we know some women are choosing to use them instead of toner on cotton wool. So with facial mists now hitting the shelves at all price points, we thought we should include them. What we discovered is that it's all down to the design as much as the skin-boosting contents, and these all performed well.

## Liz Earle Naturally Active Instant Boost Skin Tonic, £7.75/2 x 30ml

*Top Treat*

Score: 9.1/10

This is the hand-bag size spritzer version of Liz Earle's toner – an outright winner in our Toners section (see page 122), and it's scooped this, too. An alcohol- and astringent-free formula, it's based on camomile, cucumber extract and natural-source vitamin E, with a refreshing, reviving scent from rose geranium, rosewood, orange and lavender.

Comments: 'My skin felt instantly wonderfully hydrated and refreshed, invigorated and very pampered: make-up went on beautifully; fragrance lovely and fresh' • 'brilliant for hot days; grab, spritz, aaah! Instantly reviving' • 'produced a definite dewy look and softening effect' • 'skin less greasy and pores felt tighter'.

## John Masters Rose & Aloe Hydrating Mist, £21/59ml

Score: 7.6/10

Manhattan hairdresser John Masters is committed to using natural and organic ingredients – and his range has been voted 'Best Non-Food Product' at the UK's Natural Products Show. Active toning ingredients here include rose essential oil, rosewater, yeast extract (to stimulate collagen production), with antioxidants A, C, E and grapeseed extract.

Comments: 'Slightest touch produces fine spray: skin felt toned, fresh, with a slight glow' • 'definite

 *tip*

All of these products are super-refreshing if kept chilled in the fridge.

boost to skin and mind; very useful quick reviver' • 'liked it being organic and cruelty free' • 'loved this; made me feel fresh and clean; make-up looked good' • 'love, love, love the fragrance – it's a little addictive – lingers in the room'.

## Prescriptives Flight Mist, £25/125ml
**Score: 7.44/10**

The sister product to Prescriptives' famous Flight Cream, delivering 'activated water containing colloidal minerals that moisturise, awaken and energise the skin', they promise, plus cooling cucumber, aloe and caffeine.

**Comments:** 'Instantly fantastic! Really cooling, then refreshing; after that it feels almost as if you've applied a mini-slick of moisturiser' • 'skin feels lovely after this, as if I've washed my face and re-applied my make-up' • 'made my face look sort of dewy, as if my make-up had been applied with a spray gun – really nice' • 'great product: really refreshing and uplifting; my skin feels years younger'.

## Korres Orange Hydrating Face Water, £12.50/100ml
**Score: 7.35/10**

From the fast-growing Athens-based beauty brand comes a combination of orange-blossom extract, amino acids and the Amazonian plant *Mourera fluviatilis* – which blossoms during the dry season and has strong water-retaining capacity. 'Maintains skin in a moisturising microenvironment for up to six hours', say Korres.

**Comments:** 'Great for carrying round in warm conditions, or just to lift your spirits; my skin felt it had had a drink' • 'lovely uplifting orange scent' • 'skin immediately felt great, really refreshed and bright' • 'made me feel very invigorated; lovely smell – skin looked almost glowing' • 'skin felt incredibly refreshed and hydrated'.

*Beauty Steal* ✳✳ **Evian Facial Mist,** £2.95/50ml
**Score: 7.11/10**

This mist – or *brumisateur*, in French – was one of the first on the market: a mineral-water spray which Evian suggests can be used to cool down skin, remove chlorine or ocean salt, as a make-up "setter" and to rehydrate skin suffering the effects of overheated or dry office air. As it's nothing but pure Evian water, it couldn't be more natural.

**Comments:** 'Ten out of ten: nice fine mist that was fresh, cool and unfragranced – which I like; skin had no sign of redness' • 'handy size – makes me feel clean' • 'moisturised skin and brightened, gave slight dewy glow' • 'very revitalising, especially when travelling and in the car' • 'a saviour for skin in dry conditions' • 'great for centrally heated or air-conditioned atmospheres' • 'so fine that you don't have to blot dry – simply let it evaporate over your make-up'.

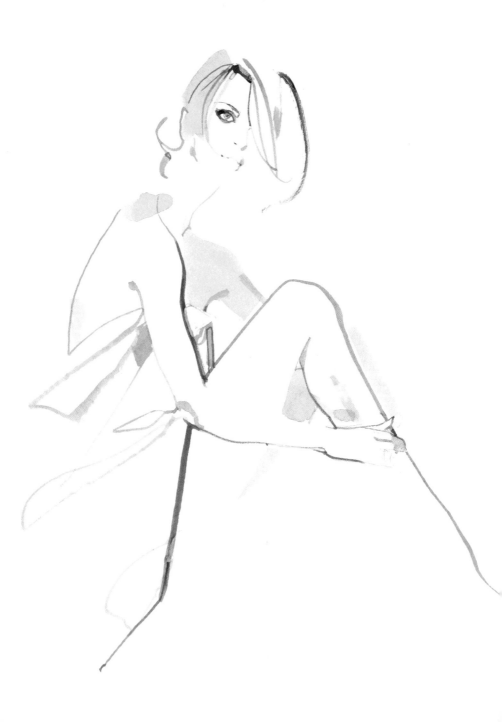

# 3

## SOS

Is your skin sending out an SOS? Is it shiny, does it break out, or do you just have a carousel's worth of excess under-eye baggage? It's time to discover the fast fixes that really work

# spot zappers

Nothing saps skin confidence more effectively than a breakout – so anything that can stop a spot in its tracks is a boon. Feedback from our testers tells us spots aren't the preserve of teenagers – one reason the beauty industry spends so much on developing products to prevent breakouts, and to help those that have erupted. Although for this book our panels of testers trialled over a dozen new products, none of them outperformed previous winners – so here's the Zit-Zapping Hall of Fame!

### Dermalogica Medicated Clearing Gel, £24.90/59ml
**Score: 8.95/10**

With the top two – very high-scoring – winners in this tough category to their credit, spot-sufferers should clearly make a beeline for Dermalogica. This is a medicated cooling gel, to be applied at night, featuring Dermalogica's anti-bacterial and anti-inflammatory Alginated Zinc Triplex complex. To help eliminate future breakouts, among the ingredients are two per per cent salicylic acid, along with vitamin A – and all our testers said that they would actually buy this.

**Comments:** 'Easy to use, quickly absorbed, clean fresh smell, and didn't sting – I used it at night and the spot was less red and sore on day one, drying out and fading on day two, almost gone on day three' • 'spots seemed noticeably less angry-looking after just one night, once I had used this' • 'calmed spots and prevented more breaking out over my whole face'.

### Dermalogica Special Clearing Booster, £30.50/30ml
**Score: 8.2/10**

Alongside the Alginated Zinc Triplex complex (see left) in this water-based gel, there's a five per cent concentration of benzoyl peroxide, plus skin-purifying and calming watercress, burdock and ivy. Applied to individual blemishes, it leaves a film on the surface, which our testers found was effective at clearing skin.

**Comments:** 'I've tried loads of spot treatments and was sure this one wouldn't deliver, but I'm a big fan now' • 'red spots and white-headed spots both healed much quicker than normally' • 'a godsend for my rather bad skin'.

### Clinique Anti-Blemish Solutions Clear Blemish Gel, £9.50/15ml
**Score: 7.79/10**

One of Clinique's top-selling products, this features pore-unblocking salicylic acid and non-irritant kola nut solution in an astringent witch hazel and alcohol base. A fast-drying clear gel, it can be worn under or over make-up.

**Comments:** 'Can be used on top of make-up and started working straight away – a whitehead disappeared' • 'my skin seemed much improved' • 'liked the rollerball; will definitely keep this near for when I feel a spot coming' • 'effective on several red, angry lumps'.

### ✳ ✳ Aesop Chamomile Concentrate Anti-Blemish Masque, £23.50/60ml
Score: 7.55/10

From an Australian natural beauty brand that we happen to love, this is a mask that targets spots. With iron oxide and montmorillite (a kind of clay), it's also loaded with anti-bacterial botanicals, and can either be left on skin under concealer or used as a rinse-off overnight treatment.

**Comments:** 'I used this on huge, bumpy, red spots and after three days, the whole area looked less angry' • 'smelt citrussy and fresh and calmly, quietly got rid of spots in two days' • 'skin felt really silky; easy to use – like a mentholy mud face pack'.

### *Beauty Steal* ✳ Body Shop Tea Tree Oil Blemish Stick, £3.50/2.5ml
Score: 7.44/10

This light, translucent gel – packed with naturally antiseptic and anti-bacterial tea tree – comes with a sponge applicator and has added sea algae to help prevent over-drying. It works out more expensive than the Dermalogica products, but is more accessibly priced, for those on a budget.

**Comments:** 'Reduced redness in an aggravated spot' • 'after the spot had dried up, there was no red mark' • 'spot healed entirely in three days – I'll buy this again' • 'handy to carry around' • 'kept the area clean and fresh'.

*tip*

● Try drinking freshly juiced carrot, celery, apple and ginger daily to build up your immune system, recommends Dr Mosaraf Ali, author of *The Integrated Health Bible*.

● Eat plenty of oily fish, carrots, avocados, pomegranates and yams.

● Preferably eat organic food whenever possible, so you don't burden your body with added synthetic chemicals; help your digestion by making sure to chew food well.

● Avoid orange and other citrus juices, which encourage inflammation of the skin.

● Also avoid yeast products, deep-fried foods, chocolates, sweets, excess salt, alcohol and coffee.

● Do remember to drink plenty of still water between meals – at least eight large glasses daily.

● For acne scarring, try pure aloe vera gel: you can even take a leaf from an aloe plant, crush it and apply the gel that oozes out with a cotton bud; also take two aloe vera capsules twice daily for three to four months.

● Another remedy for scarring is pure vitamin E oil; preferably for potency and freshness, buy capsules, prick them with a pin and put the contents on scar; rosehip oil may also help.

# oil-blotting sheets

When faces get shiny, it's tempting to powder – but that can leave make-up looking caked and unnatural. So the beauty world came up with these little sheets of 'blotting paper', which can be pressed on to make-up – or clean, oily skin – to mop up any shine. Our testers were impressed

*Top Treat*

## MAC Blot Film, £10/30 sheets
Score: 8.26/10

Larger than most of the oil-blotting papers you'll find, these are made of a special material that has been patented by 3M (who also make Post-it® Notes).

**Comments:** 'Absolutely brilliant, unbelievably absorbent, leaving skin dry, free from shine, truly matt' • 'decent-sized films that truly do the job – you only need one for the whole face' • 'fine, once I'd got over laughing at rubbing bits of balloon over my face!' • 'very effective – absorbed shine without drying the face'.

## Clinique Stay-Matte Oil-Blotting Sheets, £7.50/50 sheets
Score: 8.18/10

According to Clinique, these sheets absorb up to twice as much oil as traditional blotting papers. They come in a handy pack the size of a business card case.

**Comments:** 'Excellent product – it was very effective' • 'really good at absorbing oil; the plastic-filmy texture made it very easy to press into the crease around nose' • 'this product delivers everything it promises – eliminating shine, while leaving the skin feeling genuinely clean and free from unwanted gunge'.

*tip*

New York day spa owner Dorit Baxter counsels shiny clients to load up on foods rich in beta-carotene, such as dark green, leafy and orange fruits and vegetables. These, she says, are natural antidotes to oil overload. She also recommends avoiding caffeine. And if shine is a problem, you might like to check out our reviews of mattifying products on pages 26-7 as well.

## ❋ Space NK Oil Blotting Papers,
£8/150 sheets
**Score: 8.05/10**

From one of our favourite 'beautiques', these papers are produced from natural manila hemp pulp, making the stylish, translucent plastic pack surprisingly economical.

**Comments:** 'Thoroughly recommend these fantastic little gizmos. Very easy to use, lightweight and brilliant at doing what it says they will do' • 'no shine returned afterwards, and, surprisingly, they didn't take a shred of makeup off, just oil' • 'these were very effective at removing shine; I found them really nice to use, and only needed to use them every four hours – usually it's two' • 'removed excess oil leaving no residue, just a clean, fresh look; very convenient and portable' • 'I loved the minimalist classy packaging'.

## Smoothies' Blots,
£3.99/30 sheets
**Score: 7.6/10**

These come in a nifty little black packet, and the makers claim their oil-blotting tissues absorb three times as much as other brands.

**Comments:** 'Great texture, elegant design, no powdery residue left afterwards, and they succeeded in removing a considerable amount of shine per paper' • 'they didn't take off my make-up, which was impressive' • 'two of my friends used them and I could really see that they worked' • 'I particularly like that they can be used so discreetly' • 'shine disappeared immediately, leaving skin truly matt'.

# instant face savers

Some days, you just need a skin miracle – now! After a late night, or one spent tossing and turning, post-op, post-flu, or when skin is generally in the doldrums. So these are the 'fast fixes' that – as some of our testers put it – really are the equivalent of a facelift in a bottle

### Top Treat | Clarins Beauty Flash Balm, £22.50/50ml
**Score: 8.8/10**

Flash Balm is truly deserving of its place in the 'Beauty Hall of Fame', according to our delighted testers. Over 20 years after its launch, it is still one of Clarins's bestsellers, known as their 'Cinderella-in-a-tube' for the way it instantly plumps out lines, setting to a firming film that gives skin back its glow.

**Comments:** 'I got married recently and after little sleep was looking a less than radiant bride – this restored a nice healthy glow!' • 'I truly believe this should be every woman's beauty secret' • 'it's become one of the my must-haves – I'm not a cosmetic junkie, but this is fab' • 'my face glowed as soon as the product went on' • 'used it on combination skin – and words fail me: I look and feel wonderful – I'm 51 but it made me look 40'.

> ### tip
> Keep your instant face saver in the fridge, to maximise its face-waking power.

### Aveda Tourmaline-Charged Protecting Lotion, £35/75ml
**Score: 8.37**

Aveda generally pitch this as a longer-term, anti-ageing moisturiser – but they were confident enough about the instant benefits that the product can offer to ask us to test it in this 'instant face-saver' category. It is based on tourmaline – a crystalline, semi-precious gem which has been crushed – along with antioxidants beta-carotene, lycopene and sugar extracts, with an SPF15 chemical sunscreen, plus seven skin-refreshing pure flower and plant essences. We like the fact that it's packaged in a partly recycled tube.

**Comments:** 'I'd give this eleven out of ten – it sent my eye bags into the next millennium and it really seemed to lock in moisture and help to boost my sagging skin' • 'my skin felt very fresh after application – it soon wakes you up' • 'this was absolutely brilliant – it infused my skin with visible life and radiance, restoring moisture balance' • 'it glided on beautifully; exactly what was needed to help cheer up my winter-dull skin' • 'my skin looked even – and full of vitality' • 'after using this, my whole face felt uplifted'.

## Decléor Instant de Beauté Instant Beauty Booster, £25.50/50ml

Score: 8.22/10

Ingredients in this silky cream – which Decléor promise 'will eliminate all traces of fatigue in seconds' – include borage oil and antioxidant wheatgerm oil. If used regularly, it's claimed, it will refine and tone, improving skin texture – though our testers were asked to investigate only its immediate benefits – and is said to provide a great base for make-up. If your skin is dry, Decléor recommend that you should use your normal moisturiser over the top.

**Comments:** 'Instead of feeling 50ish, I felt 40ish – lovely' • 'like a facelift, at a fraction of the cost' • 'a fabulous boost for one's looks and confidence – like an instant facelift' • 'used it when recovering from a heavy cold and skin looked relaxed and radiant; a real find for those days when you don't feel so perky' • 'a fantastic base for make-up; I felt positively glowing by the end of the day'.

great it looks' • 'promised miracles – and delivered!' • 'saved me on New Year's Day as I'd drunk too much: should be available on prescription'.

## Jurlique Herbal Recovery Gel, £42.50/30ml

Score: 7.88/10

An all-botanical, lightweight serum from a truly natural Australian brand. (Their founder used to work for Dr Hauschka.) We have trialled this for previous books as an anti-ageing product, but this time it has done brilliantly as a quick fix. The potent botanicals and antioxidants include herbal extracts from organic roses, liquorice, marshmallow, calendula, daisy, violet, aloe, quince and camomile, plus rosehip, evening primrose, carrot, macadamia and jojoba oils. Jurlique say that it makes a great 'skin shield' – for instance, when flying.

**Comments:** 'Magical – this product makes my easily irritated skin look calm, smooth and well cared for and has people commenting on how

## Neal's Yard Remedies Zest Spritzer, £10/100ml

Score: 7.66/10

The face-waking power of this 100 per cent natural preservative-free aromatherapy spray for face, body and space is down to its combination of essential oils of lemon, bergamot and palmarosa, blended with Australian Bush Flower Essences. It was the best buy among the less expensive face-wakers and, Neal's Yard promise, its aromatherapeutic power will also 'lift you out of your mid-afternoon slump'.

**Comment:** 'Felt awake – like a slap in the face, but nicer!' • 'zesty, lifting my spirits and leaving me revived' • 'I spritzed this on bed linen, and in wardrobes, too, for a very refreshing, clean smell' • 'a wonderful pick-me-up after a bout of flu'.

# treats for tired and puffy eyes

Eyes may be the windows to our soul, but for most of us, they're often less than sparkling. So we asked our testers to trial products that claim to do away with puffiness and dark circles, and refresh tired eyes. Our testers were asked to report only on instant benefits, but many opted for a longer-term approach and noted improvements over time. But please remember these are cosmetic products, not surgery – which some testers seemed to be expecting. Somewhat to our surprise, hardly any testers reported sensitivity to these products, the majority of which are brand new launches

## Top Treat

### Elemis Eye Support, £29/30ml
**Score: 8.44/10**

Elemis's latest eye treat is a daily maintenance gel cream for line-prevention around eyes – and lips – but our testers raved about its instant depuffing and revitalising action. This pump-action product is formulated with shavegrass, to strengthen collagen and elastin, myrrh, wheatgerm and macadamia nut oils.

**Comments:** 'Ten out of ten! Eyes were brighter, refreshed, skin smoother' • 'sore, gritty, tired eyes immediately woke up and felt 110 per cent better; dark circles less noticeable' • 'specs and contacts weren't smeary or greasy; powerful effect on puffiness and creasing' • 'could apply over make-up without disturbing'.

### Shiseido The Skincare Eye Soother, £26/15ml
**Score: 8.25/10**

This gel gets its de-puffing, bag-erasing power from vitamin E and houttuynia leaves, and has crushed pearl pigments to 'bounce' light off the under-eye zone.

**Comments:** 'Good you could apply over make-up' • 'so soothing and effective at cooling

**tip** De-puff before a big night in a Turkish (steam) bath. Or try a bowl of steaming water with your head shrouded in a towel. Other old faves include cooled camomile teabags, slices of raw potato and stroking on ice cubes.

**Comments:** 'A mini-lift in a tube – reduced dark circles and puffiness, made me look wide awake' • 'lightened whole eye area, eyes brighter, skin firmer' • 'refreshing, effective on bags and an excellent make-up base' • 'a lifesaver! eyes look tight and refreshed, despite very little sleep'.

## ❋ ❋ Dr Hauschka
### Eye Solace, £18/10 x 5ml vials
Score: 7.76/10

This 'natural wonder' product has eyebright, fennel extract, woundwort, camomile and rose essential oil in a cooling lotion, which our testers unanimously found super-refreshing.

**Comments:** 'Rested my eyes and took away the strained feeling at the end of the day' • 'very cooling and refreshing: red tired eyes much clearer' • 'excellent before and after a big night out' • 'great for a pampering lazy day: ten minutes to soothe, cool and reduce redness' • 'eyes felt "alive" again'.

the skin: you need only a small amount' • 'reduced dark circles after two hours' • 'eyes were loads brighter and more awake looking – almost normal again after a late night'.

### *Beauty Steal* Champneys All-in-One Complete Eye Care, £10/15ml
Score: 8.11/10

Sneaking in as a 'Beauty Steal' for its multi-tasking abilities, this new Champneys SPF15 gel de-puffs and soothes with butcher's broom, camomile and glycerine. It has light-reflective pigments, so bags and puffiness are instantly less visible.

**Comments:** 'Better than my usual famous-name concealer for banishing dark under-eye shadows' • 'good base for make-up' • 'could be applied over make-up and made eyes look instantly brighter – I'd definitely buy this again'.

### Clarins Eye Revive Beauty Flash, £20.50/20ml
Score: 8.05/10

The new 'baby sister' to instantly face-saving Beauty Flash Balm, this rose-scented, non-greasy cream-gel, designed for tired eye emergencies rather than daily treatment, shot up our charts. It combines extracts of wheat proteins, white tea extract, vitamin K, rose and water lily extract, plus Clarins's Anti-Pollution Complex.

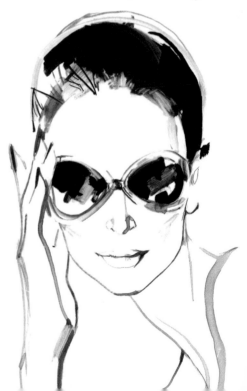

# multi-purpose balms

We love, love, love balms. And so did our 'balmy army' of testers, some of whom were balm virgins. They do everything from softening cuticles and soothing patches of chapped skin or sore lips to slicking unruly locks, setting lippie and even removing make-up and moisturising skin. Every handbag and washbag should have a pot or tube of balm for beauty emergencies and general TLC

**WE LOVE…**

We both splurge on ESPA Botanical Rescue (opposite). Jo also loves organic Balm Balm, just £2.99, fragrance-free skin magic by aromatherapist Glenda Taylor, while Sarah's all-round fave is Liz Earle's Superbalm (opposite).

## Beauty Steal — Boots Mediterranean Wonderbalm, £4.20/30ml
Score: 8.5/10

Organic sweet almond and olive oil are blended with calming sage in a dinky, portable pot. This is a true multi-purpose balm at an excellent price, according to our testers.

**Comments:** 'Brilliant as a get-all-your-bits-in-order general cream' • 'lips look glossy and well moisturised; great for heels and cuticles' • 'I have psoriasis and suffer from skin cracking behind my ears – this completely cleared it' • 'sank in quickly with no greasy residue'.

## Elizabeth Arden Eight Hour Skin Protectant, £19/50ml
Score: 8.4/10

This thick balm, often described as the 'Eighth Wonder of the Beauty World', was originally created by Elizabeth Arden for her horses' hooves. Celebrities and beauty editors often declare Eight Hour Cream their 'desert island beauty must-have'.

**Comments:** 'Excellent dry-skin quencher and nail strengthener; sorted out some psoriasis and worked miracles on my elderly father's "broken down" skin' • 'good for slicking eyebrows and on eyelashes' • 'fantastic for healing burns and scabs quickly and reducing scarring' • 'excellent for my frequently washed hands – temporarily plumped chest skin and disguised fine lines'.

## *Beauty Steal* ☀ ☀ Champneys Super Calm Rescue Balm, £5/15ml
**Score: 8.1/10**

Therapists from Champneys' spas helped create this sweet-smelling balm, which infuses sweet almond oil, cocoa butter, carnauba wax and beeswax with stress-soothing geranium, camomile and lavender essential oils.

**Comments:** 'I love this product: what more can I say!' • 'smelt lovely, and a little goes a long way' • 'my feet are much softer and smoother' • 'greatly improved my cuticles' • 'I carry this everywhere: great on lips and nails, and as a rescue product for flaky patches' • 'improved everything! I liked the reusable pot'.

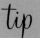 **tip** You'll be amazed how many beauty tasks you can get a balm to perform, from grooming brows to calming skin. One tester suggests: 'For dry or calloused feet, apply your chosen balm before going to bed, slip on cotton socks overnight, *et voilà!*' Sarah keeps pots by her computer, under the telly, by her bed and in her glove box and does lips, frown lines, cuticles and elbows in a few seconds.

## ☀ ☀ Liz Earle Superbalm, £13/30g
**Score: 7.9/10**

The heavenly scent as you open this pot of mega-nourishment comes from its essential oil blend of rosehip, neroli, lavender and camomile, alongside softening vitamin E and shea butter, beeswax and carnauba wax, which work to protect skin from the elements.

**Comments:** 'Gave me super soft and kissable lips with a sheen' • 'a star product! Even works on my dry frizzy hair' • 'dry patches instantly smoothed and moisturised' • 'a very little goes a very long way' • 'excellent on cuticles' • 'left me with very soft huggable elbows!'

## ☀ Nuxe Rêve de Miel® Baume des Familles, £19.50/50ml
**Score: 7.7/10**

From 'cult' French brand Nuxe – loved by skin-conscious Frenchwomen and those in the know – this generous tube is described as 'first aid skin care for the whole family', with five botanical oils, six floral waxes, shea butter and skin-calming allantoin, plus an SPF12.

**Comments:** 'A really good all-purpose cream that maxes the moisture in your skin' • 'took roughness away instantly' • 'my whole family loved it as a lip balm – my brother wants a tube of it as a Christmas present' • 'great for chaffs, red noses and unsightly dry areas' • 'worked well on my very dry feet'.

## ☀ ESPA Botanical Rescue, £30/40ml
**Score: 7.5/10**

It's pricey but several testers say they wouldn't be able to live without a tube of this rescue balm to hand, with its calming cocktail of eucalyptus, lavender, geranium, camomile and ylang-ylang oil in a base blend of shea butter with olive, sweet almond and evening primrose oils. And we're inclined to agree.

**Comments:** 'Ten out of ten for a great product: I loved it most as a lip balm' • 'my elbows have gone from crocodile skin to silk cushions' • 'the smell really makes you smile' • 'rescued my skin all over – just like it says' • 'I also used it with a face mask to intensively moisturise my face' • 'comfort and luxury all in one'.

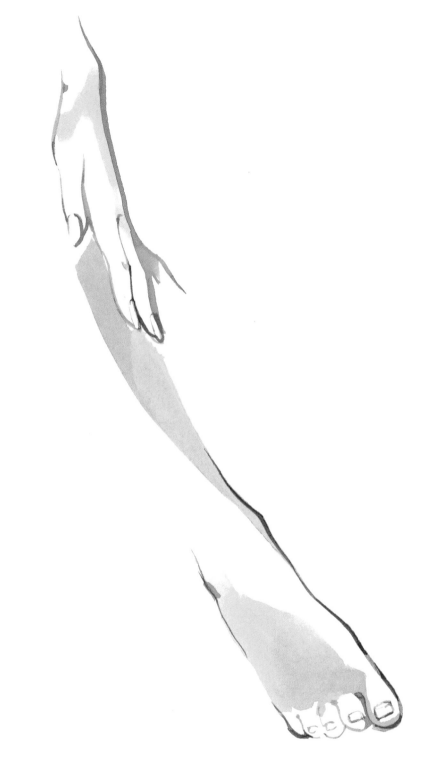

# 4

# Hands & feet

Soft, smooth hands.
Kissable feet. No more nail niggles.
The feel-good factor from elegant
extremities is undeniable –
so for everything from long-lasting
polishes to quick dries via
put-the-spring-back foot
treats, just turn the page

# long-lasting nail polishes

Chipped, worn nail polish is a grooming no-no – so a truly long-lasting polish is high on the beauty wish list of every woman who paints her nails. To test these products, our panellists were instructed not to use additional topcoat or quick-dry – and the winners, they tell us, are veritable Duracell bunnies

## tip

Polish will last longer if you don't soak your hands in a bath or long shower after you've painted them. Hot water softens the polish, encouraging peeling. If you have flaking nails, try a supplement of magnesium (see Nail Treatments tip, page 91) – take it at night and it helps you sleep, too – and diligently massage in Dr Hauschka's Neem Nail Oil, £21/30ml, twice daily.
PS: the bottle lasts for ever.

### Top Treat · Estée Lauder Pure Color Sheer Strength Nail Foundation, £12.50

**Score: 8.5/10**

Actually designed as a ridge-smoothing base coat, this makes a fabulous neutral polish worn on its own. Light-reflecting pigments minimise the appearance of ridges and imperfections. 'Satin micro mica-particles' (as Lauder describe them) help make the polish water-resistant.
**Comments:** 'Very durable – made nails look shiny and healthy; felt stronger to the touch' • 'looked great: shiny, glossy and very durable' • 'survived a range of office duties'.

### Chanel Le Vernis Nail Colour, £12

**Score: 8.25/10**

Who can resist Chanel packaging? Not us, certainly. But what impressed our testers was the staying power of this polish, which comes in a wide range of shades frequently updated to mirror catwalk trends. This has 'bioceramides', for their nail-hardening action, and the formula is free of toluene, a questionable chemical frequently found in nail polish. Every tester loved this.
**Comments:** 'Touch-dry in 60 seconds – the easiest polish to apply I've ever used' • 'it's just

starting to chip after four days – impressive, after housework and gardening!' • 'just one coat was enough to give the "I've-made-an-effort" look for work' • 'on holiday lasted a week without chipping' • 'my mother commented that her nails felt stronger after a few applications'.

## Jessica Custom Nail Colour, £7.15
**Score: 8.22/10**

This polish was created by Hollywood nail guru Jessica Vartoughian to be smooth flowing, ultra-rich and highly lustrous. The formulation incorporates vitamins A and D, to nourish the nails, so Jessica tells us.

**Comments:** 'This is the best nail varnish ever: no streaks or lines, hid ridges, one coat covered, two for stronger colour; touch dry in 30 seconds; my nails usually chip in a day – this lasted more than three' • 'lasted a very impressive seven days and I loved the natural colour – I'm breathless!' • 'I got so many compliments when I wore this: really impressed with finish and staying power'.

## Rimmel French Manicure with Lycra®, £3.99
**Score: 8.11/10**

You know what Lycra does for clothes: makes them stretchy and flexible. That's why Rimmel has incorporated Lycra into this small selection of nude polishes, which promise to deliver up to five days' 'shockproof' chip resistance.

**Comments:** 'So good: lasted four days without chipping; I'm hopeless at applying, but this was a breeze and dried so quickly I didn't have time to smudge' • 'I loved the colour and texture; reasonably priced and lasted two days without chipping; fabulously easy to apply – great brush' • 'I couldn't believe such a cheap nail polish would be so good; colour very subtle and classy; hands look instantly cared for'.

## Essie Perfect Nails, £7.50
**Score: 7.95/10**

Originally created for professionals, Essie is now very popular with those of us who like to paint our nails *chez nous*, with six fashion shades launched each season to join the 300 in the Essie range.

**Comments:** 'Easiest polish I've ever applied; went on fantastically smoothly' • 'fabulous base for a French manicure' • 'dried really quickly • 'top marks – it just didn't chip! Wore off before that' • 'good brush – and five to six days' wear'.

## OPI Nail Lacquer, £8.95
**Score: 7.66/10**

Oh, how they worship their nails in Hollywood. OPI is another range to have originated in Tinseltown – and this lacquer (which has won many beauty awards) is a celebrity fave, packed with pigments for depth of colour and cover, in a huge, fashion-inspired range of shades.

**Comments:** 'Lovely shine and richness; dried in 90 seconds, too' • 'glorious colour, good shine, excellent cover' • 'no need for top coat; lasted a good four days with typing, housework – brilliant!' • 'one coat is enough'.

# nail quick dries

We'd love to be the type of women who have time to sit around wafting our hands elegantly while waiting for our nails to dry – but we're not. So quick-dry products – sprays, oils or top coats that help stop smudging, denting and smearing – are a boon. To be honest, our testers weren't overwhelmed by these products, but these were the ones that enabled them to 'paint and go' most effectively

### China Glaze Fast Forward Top Coat, £7.50

*Top Treat*

**Score: 7.15/10**

China Glaze is a Hollywood-based brand (where manicures matter) and this paint-on top coat and quick-dry in one is said to 'penetrate and dry all layers of nail polish quickly'. Testers were actually more impressed by the professional look and long-lasting finish.

**Comments:** 'Nails felt touch-dry in five minutes (ten without the product), dry enough to get on with life in 15 minutes (40 without) – and polish lasted four days before the first chip' • 'brilliant! Normally a manicure lasts two days before the polish starts flaking off my weak nails, but four days is the new record' • 'nails looked as if I'd had a professional manicure'.

### OPI Drip Dry Lacquer Drying Drops, £11.50

**Score: 6.85/10**

Squeeze a drop of this oil on to polish and, according to OPI, 'it creates a perfectly dry,

high sheen finish within five minutes'. The drops are packed with nourishing vitamin E, jojoba and an 'Advanced Avocado Lipid Complex' to nourish your cuticles at the same time as speed-drying your manicure.

**Comments:** 'Nails felt touch-dry in ten to 15 minutes, compared to 30 minutes without using this' • 'I've recommended this to all my friends because it is *very* easy to use, and seemed to make the varnish tough and last longer – with no polish on, it treated my nails and cuticles without being oily' • 'I was really please that there was no smudging at all'.

### Creative Nails Solar Speed Dry Spray, £19.95

**Score: 6.72/10**

This spritz contains nail-conditioning jojoba, vitamin E and sweet almond oils, which also help prevent the occurrence of hangnails. Some of our panellists really loved the marzipan-y smell, too – but beware, if you are not a fan. According to Creative Nails, nail enamel should be dry one to two minutes after application of the spray.

**Comments:** 'Love it, love it, love it! Normally I hate applying top coat, but this was so easy' • 'my nails were touch dry in 60 seconds and I could carry on doing things normally within five minutes' • 'I really liked this for lots of reasons – it dried the polish quicker, smelt really fab and moisturised my cuticles' • 'I liked the spray application, which prevents overuse'.

### Rimmel Speed Dry with Lycra®, £3.99
**Score: 6.5/10**

Rimmel have incorporated Lycra® into several of their nail products to improve flexibility, elasticity and, as a result, chip-proofing. This paint-on top coat is designed to dry nails in just 60 seconds while delivering a superb, shock-proof shine.

**Comments:** 'Touch dry in under one minute, fine to carry on in 20 minutes, and the polish lasted six days before the first chip' • 'I have long nails and operate a till and keyboard, and I was amazed at the length of time it lasted' • 'by the time I'd painted the second hand and applied the top coat, the first hand was already touch dry' • 'a good-value product, which did its job and gave a lovely shine'.

## WE ♥ LOVE...

Jo occasionally plumps for Revlon Top Speed® Top Coat, £5,99/14.7ml, or Seche Vite Dry Fast Top Coat, £7.99/0.5oz, but here's our favourite DIY trick, which we both swear by: a drop of almost any kind of oil (even olive) on polish that's just touch dry makes it set fast, stops fluff ruining your manicure and is a treat for your cuticles, too.

# nail polish removers

Tired of polish removers that require elbow grease to do the job properly? So were we. So our testers got swiping, trying dozens of removers. They found some terrific formulas – and some innovative ideas – that make this beauty chore almost a pleasure. No daisies for naturalness in this chapter – the only truly 'natural' way to enhance nails is to buff them, not paint them

## tip

The art of nail polish removal is simple: soak the pad generously, then hold it over the polished nail for a few seconds to start the process of dissolving before swiping the polish away. If you just start skimming the pad over the top, it takes lots of rubbing. For more great nail tips, turn to manicure guru Leighton Denny's secrets, on pages 18-19.

### Beauty Steal — Skin Benefits Conditioning Nail Polish Remover Wipes, £1.99/15 pads

Score: 8.7/10

Cute, these: a resealable sachet of 15 individually packed acetone-free swipes, with vitamin E and aloe vera, to help prevent nails drying out.

**Comments:** 'Loved this: worked extremely well – actually gripped the polish rather than smearing it everywhere; didn't dry nails' • 'Eleven out of ten! One pad did finger and toenails; especially great on holiday' • 'removed two-week-old burgundy polish efficiently' • 'individual packaging is particularly good – you can keep one in your bag'.

### Cutex Moisture Guard Nail Polish Remover Wipes, £1.99/5 wipes

Score: 8.6/10

Featuring Cutex's Moisture Guard Formula Nail Polish Remover with Nail Whitener – designed for dry, brittle nails – these individually wrapped sachets slip neatly into a sponge bag. We haven't declared them a 'Beauty Steal' because there are only five to a pack. If you like them, it would be less wasteful to use Cutex remover itself, when not travelling.

**Comments:** 'Would definitely buy these: much easier, pleasant smell, everything removed and no residue; made cuticles softer and nails look healthy' • 'perfect for on the go' • 'easy to remove all polish with minimum of effort' • 'certainly not drying' • 'brilliant for travelling, because they have a foil wrapper – efficient at removing the thick red polish on my toes'.

### OPI Polish Remover with Aloe Vera, from £2.20/30ml

**Score: 8.37/10**

This green-tinted remover in a small plastic bottle features just a touch of acetone, a highly effective polish remover – but because acetone's drying, they've added aloe vera to counterbalance the problem. OPI recommend using this polish on either natural nails or enhancements together with their special OPI lint-free Nail Pads – although some of our testers didn't, and were still very impressed.

**Comments:** 'One application efficiently removed dark nail polish' • 'clear squeezable container made it easy to get required amount' • 'my nails look better from using this: it just does the job quickly, easily, efficiently; I wouldn't use any other remover now' • 'definitely recommend using with OPI Nail Wipes to save on product wastage'.

### girl2go Polish Off Nail Varnish Remover Wipes, £1.99/15 wipes

**Score: 8.33/10**

From girl2go's collection of mini-essentials 'for fast-lane females' – in their words – these citrus-fragranced wipes have moisturising properties to condition nails; in other words, they're oily, according to our testers.

**Comments:** 'One pad removed all the polish from my finger nails; nails felt conditioned and moisturised' • 'very effective, no unpleasant smell, ideal to take on holiday' • 'great! Removed polish quicker and better than my usual brand – one pad

did both feet; pads felt flimsy but did the job well' • 'excellent packaging, and no nail polish smell'.

### Christian Dior Nail Polish Remover, £9/50ml

**Score: 8.04/10**

In its gorgeous, very 1950s original Dior bottle, this pretty pink polish remover is one for the dressing table: a combination of acetone and water with a 'hydro-emollient' agent, to prevent whitening of nails. But at a luxury price tag…

**Comments:** 'Very gentle and effective at removing polish; no need to rub or repeat – removed polish in one go' • 'base coat, two dark lacquer coats and topcoat came off with ease and nails were in excellent condition' • 'has become my best friend' • 'despite containing acetone, smelt fragrant like face powder' • 'a truly luxury item'.

# nail treatments

The perfect nail is strong, but flexible – too-hard nails just snap off. And if you're not blessed with naturally great nails, there's a lot you can do to boost nail health, strength and resilience – as our testers discovered

**NB:** none of these works miracles overnight, so testers were asked to use them for a month or more – on just one hand, for comparison. Meanwhile, a warning: chemical treatments may eventually make nails over-hard and prone to snapping – although that won't happen with a nail oil such as Decléor's, or the creams below.

## WE LOVE...

Jo keeps a little pot of Mandarin Nail Treatment Balm, £16/45g – made by our friends at Circaroma for the fabulous spa at Pennyhill Park – on her bedside table, and at her computer is ESPA Botanical Rescue, one of the winners in our Tried & Tested multi-purpose balms category (see page 81). Sarah swears by rubbing in Dr Hauschka's Nail Neem Oil, £21/30ml, but do keep on applying it daily, even when your nails look good – or bingo, they tend to start flaking again. Or try massaging in Liz Earle's fab Superbalm, £13.50/30g.

## OPI Nail Envy, £16.50/15ml
**Score: 8.07/10**

Nail Envy – a celebrity fave rave – is now available in various strengths, but our testers were assigned the original. According to OPI, it's ideal for weak, damaged nails, and it can be used as a base coat, as a nail polish – on its own, for a clear manicure – or, for maintenance, once nails are stronger, painted on as a top coat, once a week.
**Comments:** 'Made a big difference; I'd definitely recommend it' • 'lovely clear, glossy finish; after using this for a month, my nails look rosy, healthy, buffed and smooth, with no flaking' • 'easy to use – love this; an excellent top coat too' • 'definite strengthening benefits after a week or two'.

*Beauty Steal* ## Perfect 10 Super Strength, £4.45/16ml
**Score: 7.9/10**

To help thin, weak nails, this fast-drying formula, which you apply daily to clean nails, is fortified with panthenol and a vitamin complex which they claim 'bonds with the nails instantly, helping to build stronger, healthier-looking nails with just one coat'. Most of our testers would buy it but pointed out it only worked while it was on.

**Comments:** 'The strength when applied was phenomenal and the shine was divine, but when I took it off, my nails were no better' • 'gives an acrylic-like coating; made my nails feel stronger and they appeared to grow while I used it; fine as long as I was using the product' • 'easy to apply to my weak, flaky, peeling nails, which become stronger and more flexible' • 'great staying power'.

**tip** Weak flaking nails may need a targeted supplement too, such as BioCare's Hair & Nail Complex (see page 148). Magnesium may help nails; Sarah takes BioCare Magnesium Pantothenate, £8.55/60 capsules, or Dyno-Mins Magnesium, £12.05/90 tablets.

## Crabtree & Evelyn Gardeners Nail & Cuticle Therapy, £6.95/15ml
**Score: 7.85/10**

Ubermanicurist Leighton Denny, whose nail tips we feature on pages 18-19, endorses this treatment, which has a wonderfully aromatic smell from rosemary, comfrey, clover, yarrow, calendula and lavender. He recommends using it to avoid hangnails and suggests thrice-weekly application. Over time and with diligent use, our testers found that it worked to make their nails more resilient.

**Comments:** 'Lovely product: a treat for dry and ragged cuticles; my nails seemed stronger and more flexible, and grew a little longer than usual' • 'it's really made a difference: my nails have a healthy glow, feel nourished and the whole nail and cuticle area looks in good condition; my thumbnail has been split for eight months but is growing as it should' • 'my nails are going from strength to strength – wonderful!' • 'my very dry, flaky, splitting nails were tangibly stronger'.

## ☀ ☀ Decléor Aromesssence Ongles Nail Treatment Oil, £32/15ml
**Score: 7.33/10**

As you've probably spotted from results throughout this book, Decléor have rather cornered the market in treatment oils – in this case, featuring essential oils of myrrh, lemon and parsley, in a castor/hazelnut/avocado oil base. It should be massaged into the base of nails daily – or, we suggest, nightly.

**Comments:** 'Nails tougher – flexible, not brittle – and skin conditioned' • 'nails pinker, maybe from frequent massage' • 'easy to use; left unpolished nails with a slight sheen; good at stopping flaking'.

## Crabtree & Evelyn La Source Nail & Cuticle Therapy, £6.95/15ml
**Score: 7.31/10**

We reckon the formulation of this is probably pretty similar to the Gardener's Nail & Cuticle Therapy – which scored slightly better, left – but with a different smell: a 'spa-y', marine fragrance. Whatever: Crabtree & Evelyn have obviously got this strengthening business – well, nailed.

**Comments:** 'Once I got in the habit of using it regularly, I noticed a real difference: nails much longer, and didn't split nearly as much' • 'nails looked healthier, were less brittle and could bend more without usual breaking and splitting; kept cuticles and surrounding skin nice and soft, well moisturised; a lovely product overall' • 'nails seem stronger, more flexible – not brittle at all now, and a huge improvement to the skin around nails; liked the light fragrance'.

# hand creams

One of our best nuggets of beauty advice is to leave a tube or bottle of hand cream next to every set of taps in your house – and one on your desk, and bedside table, too. These choices are rich and restorative – but they also sink in quickly enough to let you get on with life

## WE ♥ LOVE…

The soap on trains is super-drying and, since we live at opposite ends of England, we can acquire sandpaper hands by the time we meet in London. We're both huge fans of Liz Earle Naturally Active Hand Repair, £7.75/50ml; the 'mini' size, £7.75/15ml duo, is just perfect for popping in a handbag.

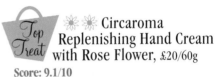

### ✽ ✽ Circaroma Replenishing Hand Cream with Rose Flower, £20/60g

**Score: 9.1/10**

A truly outstanding result for this natural cream from a tiny British aromatherapy brand (which will ship worldwide). All the products are virtually handmade, in small batches. This is based on organic rose water, rose attar, geranium and ultra-moisturising shea butter.

**Comments:** 'Smells fantastic – real rose scent, not synthetic' • 'very good on dryness, nails and cuticles, and seemed to have a whitening effect' • 'silky feel, sank in right away – a real treat' • 'my hands look younger and brighter – the best hand cream I've ever used' • 'scar on the back of my hand less noticeable – my hands are soft as cashmere and blissed out'.

### Christian Dior Mains Protective Nourishing Crème for Hands SPF8, £11.50/75ml

**Score: 8.8/10**

Christian Dior say this should 'wrap hands in a voluptuous, protective cocoon', with its ceramide-rich moisturising complex. It's designed to sink in swiftly, leaving hands velvety – and there's an SPF8, for moderate sun protection.

**Comments:** 'Skin felt velvet smooth immediately' • 'smells gorgeous; after a week, improvements were visible, particularly on my cuticles' • 'my skin looked fresh and young after using this' • 'elegantly packaged; and a little goes a long way' • 'a slight sheen on hands improved appearance of skin; noticed a good conditioning effect on cuticles'.

## ❋ ❋ Jurlique Lavender Hand Cream, £15.25/40ml
**Score: 8.77/10**

Alongside soothing lavender, this rich but non-greasy cream features rose, calendula, chamomile, honey, soya lecithin, macadamia nut oil and aloe among its ingredients.

**Comments:** 'Very hydrating – and I have the driest hands in the world' • 'can't stop looking at my hands – they appear ten years younger' • 'divine fragrance' • 'my daughter – who is a nursery nurse and prone to dry, sore hands – liked this very much as well' • 'it also made my elbows soft'.

## *Beauty Steal* Sainsbury's Active: Naturals Lavender & White Tea Hand and Nail Cream, £1.99/75ml
**Score: 8.55/10**

Throw this flip-top tube in your supermarket trolley alongside the frozen peas and, say our testers, you won't be disappointed. It's from the exclusive-to-Sainsbury's range containing 'food-based natural ingredients'.

**Comments:** 'this is really excellent for dry hands' • 'pleasing mildly herbal fragrance; nails a little pinker, hands well moisturised' • 'I didn't believe a budget hand cream could be so good – this one is a real find' • 'my hands are very smooth and soft, and nails less brittle, with soft cuticles' • 'my husband also liked this product'.

# feet treats

We believe happy feet make a happy woman – have you ever noticed the pinched expression of a woman with too-tight shoes? Packed with ingredients to invigorate and also moisturise, these creams and lotions are almost as refreshing as lying down with your feet up

Though our testers tried quite a few new foot-reviving products, when it comes to putting the spring back in a girl's step, none outperformed these true 'Beauty Oscars', which we tested for *The 21st Century Beauty Bible.*

## Aveda Foot Relief,
from £5/40ml
Score: 8.8/10

Cooling and invigorating, this soothing cream is 'designed to nourish the roughest, toughest feet', Aveda promise, while the swiftly absorbed plant oils and fruit acids soften calluses and rough patches. The sense-waking smell? That's down to deodorising lavender and rosemary.

**Comments:** 'Really, really good refreshing smell: feet were instantly tingly and less achey and sore' • 'needed a lot of rubbing in, which helped sore points' • 'considerably improved the cracks on my feet' • 'even my bunions are less painful and red after this' • the best I've ever used – send up

Fred Astaire please!' • 'I'm on my feet all day and they didn't throb as much with this' • 'reduced tenderness after wearing high heels; used on legs it took away that heavy feeling'.

## Weleda
Foot Balm, £4.95/75ml
Score: 8/10

A great-value foot-saver from a small health company with an outstanding natural heritage, which grows its herbs biodynamically. It's totally free of synthetic ingredients and features antiseptic calendula, disinfectant/anti-fungal lavender, rosemary and myrrh, along with invigorating rosemary and zingy sweet orange. Weleda tell us it works as an antiperspirant deodorant for sweaty feet, too.

**Comments:** 'I loved this – it absorbed really fast, leaving no greasy residue' • 'it made me feel as if I had new feet – reviving and refreshing' • 'loved the smell: uplifting, sharpish, non-cloying' • 'my feet felt lighter' • 'I liked the fact you could put on tights immediately after applying this'.

## L'Occitane Shea Butter
## Foot Cream, £14/150ml

**Score: 8/10**

This rich, lavender-scented cream is packed with 20 per cent shea butter, a legendary skin-softener, together with anti-inflammatory arnica and – so L'Occitane tell us – can be smoothed on over tights. Several testers reckoned it rated it as a hand cream, too.

**Comments:** 'Heaven after a hard day; delicious, refreshing smell for feet – lavender, rosemary, mint' • 'this one was the best for hard skin on heels and under toes' • 'I got immediate relief and felt definite improvement to post-high-heels ache' • 'this product was pretty perfect – and a little went a long way' • 'I can't live without this; great for long-haul flights to banish swollen ankles and heavy legs'.

## Crabtree & Evelyn
## Foot & Leg Therapy with
## Peppermint Oil, £10.50/100g

**Score: 7.88/10**

A light, creamy lotion based on shea butter with a jolt of peppermint oil, this oil aims to leave your feet feeling fresh, tingly and rejuvenated within minutes of application. The product scored highly with testers who had medical conditions, including varicose veins and – in one case – deep vein thrombosis.

**Comments:** 'The fresh cooling feeling I got from this was wonderful and lasted a long time' • 'experienced an instant refreshing feeling that made feet comfortable and really took the heat out and the tired ache away' • 'it helped to soothe the soreness and tenderness that my legs suffer from periodically' • 'I have weak veins owing to deep vein thrombosis and found that this eased the ache in my bad leg, and the feeling of tiredness in legs and feet'.

### WE ♥ LOVE…

Feet are highly absorbent and anything that you put on them is swiftly taken into the bloodstream, so – to make sure she knows exactly what is going in – Jo makes her own peppermint foot balm from her book, *The Ultimate Natural Beauty Book* (Kyle Cathie, £14.99), based on sweet almond and avocado oils with lots of zingy mint. Her biggest 'foot treat' of all, though, is a 'medi-pedi' with the incredibly talented Bastien Gonzalez in London who whisks away every atom of hard skin (£110). Sarah is equally meticulous about treating her feet: creaming is much better for them than daily buffing – do that once a week only, say experts. Currently, she likes Decléor's aromatic Beauté des Pieds Comfort Foot Cream, £15/50ml, and Barefoot Botanicals SOS Foot Rescue Balm, £9.95/50g. She aims for three-monthly sessions with podiatrists, and just revels in the Crème de la Mer Ultimate Foot Treatment, £50 for one hour, available at the Urban Retreat at Harrods: no varnish is used, but your toenails are buffed to a perfect shine with a diamond file.

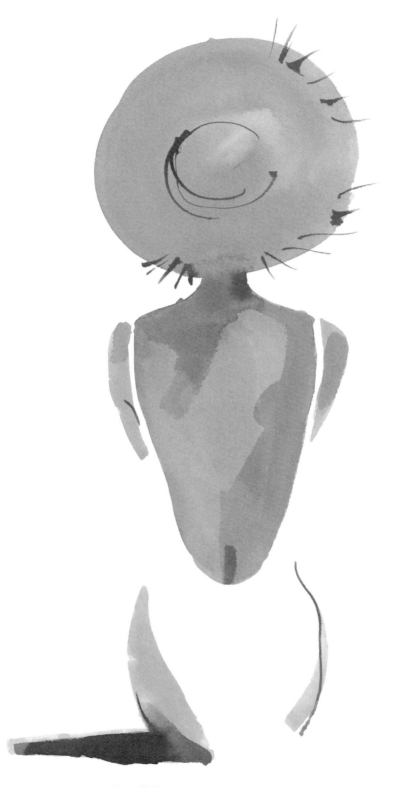

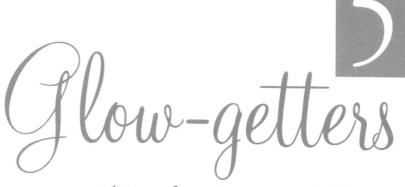

# 5

# Glow-getters

A hint of tan is a mood-lifter –
whether it's real or fake. But which
of the SPFs are really worth
stashing in your beach bag? Or the
can't-tell-it-from-Copacabana
fake tans? Our testers were
transformed into golden goddesses,
to bring you the answers

# bronzers

Whoosh! With just a touch of a great bronzer, complexions can go from drab to fab, pasty to sunkissed. But not all bronzers are created equal – so if you're looking for a version that's going to deliver a subtle glow rather than lurid stripes, listen to what our testers have to say

## WE LOVE...

The number one top scorer here, also in the lightest 'Toundra' shade, is Jo's all-time favourite bronzer – she often uses it in place of blusher, because it doesn't highlight the redness in her cheeks the way some pinky tone blushers do. Sarah's quite bronzy already, what with horses and gardens and boats...

### Top Treat

### Chanel Irréele Soleil, £22.50
**Score: 8.72/10**

A pressed powder bronzer with a 'quilted' effect – the bronzer itself looks like a Chanel handbag! – this fine blend of silica, nylon reflective pigments and vitamin E also contains light-reflecting pigments to soften the appearance of fine lines and blemishes. In a choice of three shades – our testers tried Toundra – it comes in a wide-mirrored Chanel compact. There's also quite a useful-sized brush – though you'll get better results with a big bronzing brush of your own.

**Comments:** 'Blended evenly, gave me a very natural, healthy glow' • 'loved the iridescent finish, gave a bloom over foundation and worked as well over bare skin – and, as always, Chanel packaging is lovely' • 'bronzers can look too orange but this is definitely subtle, yet still gave a healthy glow usually acquired by tanning – didn't look ageing, as with other products' • 'didn't sink into and aggravate lines; lasted about six to seven hours' • 'merged with skin to enhance it, not drying at all, like a light, soft veil of colour'.

### Ultraglow Complexsun UV Demi-Matte Bronzing Powder, £12.50
Score: 8.6/10

Some women want to shimmer in the sun, while others want to stay perfectly matt – which is why

Ultraglow created this soft, matt powder bronzer. Our testers were sent the matching powder brush, £10, which clearly makes for a can't-tell-it-from-real effect. There's a tiny bit of sun protection in there – SPF5 – but don't rely on it to do much.

**Comments:** 'This is fab; very versatile, worked well as a pick-me-up over my normal make-up, or instead of blusher' • 'colour was very scary, but looked superb on; skin looked *so* healthy' • 'looked as if I'd been in the sun all day' • 'brushed on evenly and smoothly' • 'a blusher brush was on my "to buy" list and this one fits the bill beautifully' • 'effect lasted ages; didn't need to retouch all day'.

### ☀ Origins Sunny Disposition, £15
**Score: 8.57/10**

This is a twist-up stick version of Sunny Disposition, which in its liquid format also scored highly as a three-in-one product for cheeks, eyes and lips (see page 39). This one glides on your face to give a 'sexy, sultry sheen', so Origins promise, adding that it shouldn't streak, crease or fade. Vitamin E offers antioxidant protection, while lecithin and aloe soften and smooth skin.

**Comments:** 'Very light and delicate; added a healthy glow rather than a made-up look; I used it as blusher, eye shadow and lipstick and was very pleased with the effect' • 'a couple of gentle strokes on my cheeks gave the colour I needed – for six hours; and this little gem melded perfectly with any foundation' • 'every make-up bag should have one: actually every handbag should have one instead of a make-up bag; it's gorgeous, simple, effective – stunning!'

### ☀ ☀ Dr Hauschka Bronzing Powder, £20
**Score: 8/10**

Dr Hauschka tell us that their all-natural bronzing powder is created 'using a caring combination of

**tip** Our friend and make-up guru Bobbi Brown advises that oily skins and bronzers may not get on: 'If you have oily skin, you may have to forgo the pleasure of bronzer, as oily skin can turn bronzers orange.' You won't know until you try, so experiment in-store with a 'tester', and see for yourself.

medicinal plant extracts', including witch hazel and sage, to combat skin impurities. It also has a touch of silk, which accounts for its softness.

**Comments:** 'Ten out of ten – the best bronzing powder ever. Glided on and looked totally natural; gave skin a luminescent glow, as if you'd been in the sun for a couple of days' • 'worked beautifully with mascara and lip gloss: reapplied a couple of times during the day – not sure it was necessary, I just loved it so much' • 'lovely, fine, silky powder; did not rub off on to clothes when getting dressed'.

### M&S Autograph Bronzing Powder, £12
**Score: 7.56/10**

This multi-purpose compact features both a matt powder and a cream formula shimmer – the cream shimmer can be used to highlight cheekbones or under the eyebrow, to 'lift' the eyes, they suggest. There are two shades: our testers were allocated 'Sunkissed'.

**Comments:** 'The concept of two powders is brilliantly versatile; the matt blends into my make-up while the shimmer sits on top' • 'great using the matt over tinted moisturiser for a subtle daytime look, then turning day into evening make-up with the shimmer' • 'lovely sunkissed look: I'm extremely pleased with the quality'.

# facial self-tanners

These are the safe alternatives to a real tan, if you don't want to end up with a face like the Sahara – a quantum leap from the early self-tanners, leaving skin 22-carat gold, rather than 22-carrot orange. And the technology's improving all the time

I n fact, the science of self-tanning moves on so fast that many companies replace their selection almost every year – which means one of our previous high-scorers has since been discontinued, making room for Rimmel's budget-priced offering to enter the ranking.

**Top Treat**

## Clarins Radiance-Plus Self-Tanning Cream Gel, £22.50/50ml

**Score: 8.13/10**

This clever innovation – a daily moisturiser combined with a dash of self-tanner – comes in the form of a light lotion, boasting skin-boosting vitamins, skin-softening kiwi and extract of a plant called *Larrea divaricata*, said to slow down the natural shedding of skin cells. With the pleasant fragrance its makers claim, this took around four hours to develop a really natural 'I've been in the sun' golden glow, which then lasted for around two to three days. Clarins call it 'a weekend away in a bottle'.

**Comments:** 'This product had a nice, light, easily spreadable texture' • 'didn't need make-up after putting this on – just concealer on thread veins' • 'lovely product which left me with a glowing colour – and no tide marks' • 'gave a really natural sunkissed colour – and without any burnt-cookie smell; I love it!'

## WE ♥ LOVE...

Jo agrees wholeheartedly with our testers and you'll find Clarins Radiance-Plus Self-Tanning Cream Gel (see right) on her bathroom shelf throughout the summer months; she uses it every few days and has been known to mix half and half with Estée Lauder DayWear Plus Multi Protection Antioxidant Moisturizer SPF15 Sheer Tint Release Formula. Being outside year round, Sarah doesn't need one of these!

## Lancôme Flash Bronzer Instant Bronze Glow for the Face, £18/50ml
Score: 7.78/10

Tinted pigments and light-reflecting pigments in this vitamin-enriched cream deliver an instant sun-kissed look – so you can see where you've put it – while you wait for the tan to develop. This version's designed for darker complexions; fair skins should opt instead for the Instant Golden Glow, which has a lower concentration of the active self-tanning ingredient (DHA).

**Comments:** 'After 45 minutes I had a golden glow; I loved everything about this – the smell, texture, colour and the tiny shimmering light-reflective particles' • 'great for winter wanness – turns it into a healthy glow' • 'loved the creaminess' • 'if used daily, colour builds up naturally and gradually' • 'evened out skintone, improved the texture of my skin'.

## Phytomer Bronze Perfect, £14/50ml
Score: 7.57/10

Has a 'helioprotect' complex – with allegedly anti-ageing and anti-inflammatory properties – plus nourishing oil of apricot. There's a low level of sun protection, though this remains active only immediately after application.

**Comments:** 'Effective and totally natural-looking' • 'colour was excellent' • 'great – no stickiness, no shine, natural and even-looking colour' • 'nice, healthy glow still visible after seven days' • 'natural colour; left skin feeling very moisturised'.

## Ambre Solaire No Streaks Bronzer Self-Tan Wipes, £1.39 each
Score: 7.4/10

Though they're inexpensive, we've decided these aren't truly a 'Beauty Steal' because they're one-use wipes that would prove pricy, if used all the time. Nevertheless, our testers found them a

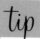

To rid yourself of reverse racoon eyes, mix a few drops of self-tanner with eye cream and dab the concoction over pale circles. The point is not to match the light skin to the dark, but to at least make the demarcation line a little less obvious.

nifty way of giving a glow to face, neck and chest – the area 50 per cent of glow-getters focus on. They feature vitamin E and apricot extract.

**Comments:** 'Excellent for a quick fix, very subtle' • 'my skin looked natural, not heavily tanned or fake' • 'easy to keep in your handbag' • 'very slight orangey smell, pleasant not synthetic'.

##  Rimmel Sunshimmer Fresh Face & Body Bronzer Self-Tan Gel, £6.99/125ml
Score: 7.27/10

A clear gel formulation that does double duty, gliding on to face and body, 'developing into a deep tan within one hour', so Rimmel declare – which means one less product cluttering up the bathroom shelf. Testers all liked it, especially for the price, and would use it all over.

**Comments:** 'Much better than other cheaper brands – almost as good as Estée Lauder; no chemical after smell, I will definitely buy and use it' • 'very good: no horrid fake tan smell at all, gel texture is easy to spread, blends in evenly; took about three hours to develop to a healthy natural glow, lasted two days' • 'very natural, even, golden colour, gave me a lift' • 'left a smooth silky finish' • 'I was pleasantly surprised – don't be put off by the "cheap" make – it's very good'.

# body self-tanners

These are a godsend at the beginning of summer – when the opaque tights get packed away – on holiday, and any time we're feeling pasty. We're often told that the only safe tan is a fake tan – so trust us, and our testers: there are some great fakes out there

**tip** If you're naturally pale and a self-tanner scaredy-cat, try mixing half and half with your regular body lotion. Blend the two together the palm of your hand, and massage in well, swiping areas like heels, toes and knees very lightly with a damp cloth afterwards to prevent build-up in those areas.

*Top Treat* **Lancaster Self Tan Silk Bronze Moisturizing Milk SPF6, £17.50/125ml**
Score: 8.77/10

This one-hour golden wonder uses a speeded-up version of DHA – the self-tanning ingredient – plus sweet orange to naturally boost skin's melanin, with watermelon and pineapple extracts to moisturise and exfoliate skin. Testers trialled the Medium shade and commented this gave a sun-kissed effect; for deeper colour you need to re-apply – or choose the Intense version.
**Comments:** 'I loved it, everything worked – colour, texture, smell and the results were great on my body – and my face' • 'excellent colour: the best fake tan I've used' • 'only had to stay undressed for a few minutes' • 'I like the slow build-up of colour; easy for first-timers' • 'harder to apply than a colourless product, but no coloured layer to rub off on clothes – an advantage!'.

## St. Tropez Whipped Mousse, £20/4oz
Score: 8.7/10

From the brand loved by stars, this super-speedy mousse dries in 60 seconds. It's 'self-adjusting' to your skintone, St. Trop promise – adding that the addition of aloe leaf and fruit acids helps achieve 'the richest, longest-lasting tan possible'.
**Comments:** 'I left it overnight and by morning I was a lovely golden brown – non-streaky and realistic' • 'subtle, sweet smelling, thick but easy

to spread and fast absorbed' • 'I felt safe sitting on my sofa after 20 minutes' • 'when I looked at myself in the shower after using this I immediately got that post-sunbathing "feel-good" factor'.

## L'Oréal Sublime Bronze Instant Tan, £10.99/30ml
**Score: 8.25/10**

This is designed for faces, in fact, but owing to the fact that the text on this product is ambiguous, to say the least, we admit we boobed by trialling it in this category. The good news is it did really well! We can't award it a 'Beauty Steal' tag because, of course, you'd need quite a lot to do your legs and/or body. Whatever: it's a facial self-tanning gel-like lotion in a dual pump, combining an instant tint, so you can see where you've applied it, and a self-tanning lotion with built-in AHAs, to exfoliate. But it clearly works jolly well on bodies.

**Comments:** 'Very realistic, natural colour, gives skin a hint of a golden glow after one application; very convincing: great product' • 'lots of friends have commented' • 'I now have a nice golden stomach instead of a pale one' • 'great product for legs' • 'very nice smell, which faded in a day, sinks into skin brilliantly; waited for about ten minutes before getting dressed' • 'very natural sunkissed colour; you don't need a lot, because it spreads very easily'.

## Ambre Solaire Gloss Bronzer, £8.99/125ml
**Score: 7.91/10**

This winner was formerly known as 'Instant Shimmer Bronzer'. The formulation is still lightly tinted – so no missed spots – prettily shimmery, and develops in just one hour.

**Comments:** 'Very natural colour lasted four days' • 'pleasant chocolatey smell; lovely smooth texture' • 'immediate colour, with an attractive shimmer – and top marks for clear instructions' • 'good subtle colour, easy to build up gradually'.

## Origins Great Pretender, £13.50/150ml
**Score: 7.88/10**

You can see exactly where you've put this tinted shimmery body gel, which has a significant proportion of natural ingredients, including sugars and vegetable-derived glycerine, infused with summery-scented essential oils of peppermint, orange and rosemary.

**Comments:** 'This product was absorbed into the skin very quickly' • 'very nice peppermint smell' • 'after using this I was pleasantly surprised by the nice golden-brown result' • 'lovely shimmery particles which were great for evenings out – didn't last after initial application' • 'appearance stays even over days'.

# instant leg tints

Our grandmothers used cold tea to dye their legs – so we thank our lucky stars to be living in the 21st century, when there's a new crop of sunless tanning products that deliver an instant glow – which you can wash off later

We think these are going to be HUGE: tans-in-a-flash, which tint pasty limbs immediately, and are free from that 'biscuit-tin' smell that's the signature of so many self-tanners. Our golden goddesses tried around a dozen of these body bronzers, and there are definitely some dodgy versions out there that will leave you decidedly carroty – or, in the case of one that Jo tried recently, with legs that looked like salamis!

Testers were asked particularly to assess budge- and smudge-proofness; in fact, although none of the winning products did come off on clothes or pale sofas, or run in the rain, our testers still worried they might.

While none scored universally high marks, all earned some glowing (oops!) praise from our testers. Like Marmite, perhaps, these are love-'em-or-hate-'em products, but we expect to see many more of them launched in the future – and of course, we'll test those, too.

## WE LOVE…

Sadly, Guerlain long ago discontinued Jo's favourite Terracotta liquid bronzer, which was nothing short of miraculous; she occasionally resorts to Prescriptives Sun Sheen Body Tint, £25/125ml, in shorter-skirt emergencies. She also sometimes just rubs tinted moisturiser into pre-moisturised legs. Sarah souses hers in DuWop's moisturising non-rub-off body make-up, Revolotion, £15.95/153g, which comes in light, medium or dark, with a sun barrier of SPF15.

*Top Treat*

### BeneFit Jiffy Tan, £17.50/200ml
**Score: 7.28/10**
We're all for beauty ranges that don't take themselves too seriously. Jiffy Tan is from BeneFit's new Wonderbod range – which also includes a 'flab-fighting' Jiggle Gel – and, they say, 'is engineered to go on evenly and stay put.' They suggest lightly blending this caramel bronze

lotion on to bare skin, claiming that it adjusts to all skintones for a natural-looking tan.

**Comments:** 'The best instant tan I've used: gave me a beautiful bronzed colour, with a bit of sparkle' • 'good quick-fix effect – and I'm useless at applying fake tan' • 'sank in quickly and legs were moisturised too' • 'didn't rub off on my clothes' • 'perfect colour, doesn't change or fade like fake tan; lovely citrussy smell' • 'only had to wait five minutes before it was safe to wear clothes' • 'this is very nice; also if the results are streaky, you can wash off and have another go'.

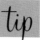

As with self-tan products, instant bronzers deliver a much more realistic, just-got-back-from-vacation glow if limbs are exfoliated and well moisturised first. In a perfect world, exfoliate, apply body lotion, wait ten minutes, then smooth on your bronzer.

## Sally Hansen Airbrush Legs, £9.95/85g
**Score: 7.05/10**

'A unique spray-on make-up for legs' is how Sally Hansen describes this aerosol, in four shades, from Light Glow to Deep Glow, so you can match your skintone. The formula, they tell us, is designed to cover up spider veins, blemishes and freckles.

**Comments:** 'Very happy to use instead of fake tan; I liked the results – good colour for light coverage' • 'really natural colour' • 'useful for top-ups on holiday' • 'washed off easily with soap or shower gel' • 'can spray upside down for backs of legs' • 'good for wearing skirts in summer' • 'didn't smudge or rub off'.

## Sexy Hair Concepts Sex Symbol Aerotan, £15.45/150ml
**Score: 6.83**

Sexy Hair Concepts promise this 'won't smear, slide, streak or sweat off', and is as good for faces as it is for legs. They also say this aerosol product can be spread thinly for a light result, or sprayed on more thickly 'for a straight-off-Copacabana sheen'. Now for our testers' thoughts...

**Comments:** 'Perfect if you had to rush in and tan, and rush out again, as it's odourless and dries so quickly; looked fantastic, with no streaks' • 'pretty

natural looking colour, with a slight shimmer' • 'colour came off easily with soap, but not with water alone – a good thing' • 'gave me a lovely glow – no trace of that horrible "I've been Tangoed" fake tan look' • 'sank in very quickly, as soon as it was blended in – no residue or film'.

## No 7 Smooth on Bronzer, £10.50/200ml
**Score: 6.33/10**

Smooth this all over, suggest Boots, 'for an instant hint of sun-kissed colour'. It features cooling, soothing, watermelon extract. The price isn't exactly peanuts, but it's the least expensive of the temporary body bronzers we trialled that scored well enough to be included.

**Comments:** 'Love wash-off tans! So convenient and perfect for lazy girls; this just took the edge off my paleness and makes me look much healthier' • 'easy to apply and blend; I would use it as an emergency product if I didn't have time to apply fake tan' • 'my usual shower gel removed it' • 'covered skin well and gave a slight flattering sheen, didn't streak in an April shower or fade all day' • 'very good as a quick fix; sank in and dried quickly – very impressive' • 'does not streak, does not smell, isn't greasy, dries instantly and colour is subtle – not remotely orange'.

# spf15 facial suncare

If you want to avoid the face-like-a-leather-handbag look in years to come, your greatest ally on vacation is a facial sunscreen, diligently applied. Dermatologists recommend nothing lower than an SPF15, because a tan today equals wrinkles in the future

It proved impossible to trial all the different levels of facial protection now on the market, so we took the experts' advice and opted for SPF15. We asked our many panels of ten testers to report on the texture, fragrance, how well the product sinks in, but – as with body SPFs – we didn't have the resources to clinically assess protection levels. As with SPF15 Moisturisers (pages 112-3), we asked companies whether their sunscreen was chemical or physical, and whether it protected against UVA and B. It's up to you to choose an SPF that works for you: we'd recommend SPF25 for paler complexions; certainly, within many ranges you'll find a higher SPF alongside factor 15s. But whatever you choose, use it, reapply during the day – and expose your face as little as possible, if you care about ageing. Some of the SPFs here can be used on the body, too – cutting down on the number of products you have to lug to the pool/beach.

## WE LOVE…

As with body suncare, Jo looks for chemical-free options: Liz Earle Naturally Active Botanical Sun Shade SPF24, £15/75ml, and Dr Hauschka Sunscreen Cream for Children, £14/100ml, which offers a higher level of protection for her English-rose colouring. Sarah uses Liz Earle, too, and also ZO1 Facial Daywear Moisturising Lotion SPF30+, £24.50/50ml, based on zinc oxide, possibly the most effective physical barrier.

 **Top Treat** Shiseido Sun Protection Lotion SPF15, £20/150ml
Score: 8.33/10

Shiseido's advanced suncare offers what they call a 'Dual Sun Protection system', a chemical barrier against UVA and UVB. This lightweight sinks-in-fast lotion doubles as body suncare.
**Comments:** 'Lovely product; preferred it to my normal sun prep' • 'went on like a moisturiser; overall it's like a body cream, not like a typical sun

cream' • 'lovely velvety texture' • 'loved the fresh floral fragrance – definite summer buy' • 'was very water resistant and protection seemed to last a long time' • 'quick and easy to apply, so am more likely to reapply regularly in the sun'.

Always apply sunscreen half an hour or more before heading for the beach – otherwise, by the time you've found a sun lounger or chosen your spot on the sand, you may already have started to burn.

## Sisley Botanical Facial Sun Cream SPF15, £75/40ml
### Score 8.11/10
Definitely priced for vacationers who can afford St Barth's or St-Trop, this thick, matt-finish cream has a synthetic chemical UVA/B filter, combined with plant extracts and essential oils to strengthen skin against damage, plus an ingredient called KVF90, which Sisley trumpet as 'the only known anti-skin cancer ingredient'.

**Comments:** 'I'm raving to all my friends about this: felt just like a face lotion; in fact, I swapped my second layer of moisturiser for this' • 'I'm now converted to using this daily as a moisturiser, and an excellent base for make-up' • 'blended in straight away and left skin instantly soft'.

## Lancôme Soleil Icy Tubes Ultra-Cooling Sun Protection Gel for Face & Body, £18/150ml
### Score: 8.05/10
Stick Icy Tubes Gel in your fridge, recommend Lancôme, and it'll feel super-cooling and icy fresh on the skin. Fruitily fragranced, Icy Tubes features antioxidant vitamins – and contains L'Oréal's patented Mexoryl chemical UVA/UVB sun filters.

**Comments:** 'The most pleasant sunscreen to apply I've ever tried – cooling even if you don't store it in the fridge; gave skin a nice dewy sheen, no hint of stickiness' • 'sank straight into skin, absorbed beautifully, made skin silky, smooth and soft' • 'lovely, fruity fragrance, very summery – enough to make you reapply it every 15 minutes' • 'didn't need fragrance as well – a bonus!'.

## Clinique City Block Sheer Oil-Free Daily Face Protector SPF15, £12/40ml
### Score: 8.05/10
This lightweight titanium and zinc-based formula guards against UVA and UVB and, because it's based on a physical (chemical-free) sunscreen – zinc oxide and titanium dioxide – this should be a good choice for sensitive skins.

**Comments:** 'Very light and smooth; sank in really quickly; kept moisture in skin even after a long day outdoors; no sun lotion smell or greasy feeling' • 'seems to help keep environmental grime off the skin' • 'convenient size for a handbag'.

## L'Oréal Solar Expertise Active Anti-Wrinkle Sun Cream SPF15, £10/75ml
### Score: 7.56/10
Formulations in this range are enriched with Activa-Cell™, which, say L'Oréal, 'stimulates the skin's natural self-repair and defence mechanisms'. This is UVA/UVB protective, with the same chemical sun filters you find in Lancôme.

**Comments:** 'Very moisturising; a small amount went a long way' • 'my fair skin didn't burn, as it would usually' • 'liked the fresh, slightly lemony smell' • 'thick but easy to apply, didn't need much rubbing in' • 'skin felt really moist but not greasy' • 'effective on a very hot day: liked this very much'.

# spf15 body suncare

Dermatologists advise that you should never go below an SPF15 when you're sunbathing: bodies will still tan, the tan will last for longer – and your skin will thank you for it. Based on our testers' opinions, here are the body products that deserve their place in the sun

We asked our testers to report on how well the creams smoothed in, the texture, fragrance and pleasure factor – but, to be fair, with far-flung testers, multiple skintones and variable weather, it was impossible to ask them about the efficiency of protection offered. The bottom line, though, is that if a product is nice to use, you're more likely to enjoy applying it – which will encourage you to be diligent about protection. In a perfect world, all sun creams would offer protection against UVA rays as well as burning UVB – and to help you identify those that do, we've done the homework for you.

## WE LOVE…

Jo is allergic to many chemical sunscreens, so she sticks to those with mineral-derived 'physical' sunblocks – titanium dioxide and zinc oxide – particularly **Liz Earle Naturally Active Sun Shade SPF15** (opposite), and **Dr Hauschka Sunscreen Cream, £13/100ml**. Sarah uses **Z01**, an Australian brand which is based on nano-particles of zinc oxide.

## Top Treat

### Biotherm Sunfitness SPF15 Waterproof Sport Spray, £15/150ml

**Score: 8/10**

Sand proof, salt proof, water proof, perspiration proof – those are the promises that Biotherm, a L'Oréal brand newish to the UK, make for this non-pore-blocking spray, which has a chemical UVA/UVB filter. A cocktail of minerals and 'pure extract of thermal plankton' help to regenerate and soothe skin.

**Comments:** 'Very light and easily absorbed; effective moisturiser, too – really efficient during sport, because it did not make me sweat overly, like most other products' • 'will definitely use sprays in the future, as so easy to apply' • 'very nice refreshing smell; feels fantastic on skin, very moisturising and soft – luxurious' • 'like it being so light, rather than greasy cream or oil'.

## Dermalogica Full Spectrum Block SPF15, £18.20/118ml
**Score: 7.8/10**

With a chemical sunscreen to shield against UVA, UVB and infrared rays, this cream has an anti-inflammatory herbal base of mint, with antioxidant grapeseed and green tea. Plant-derived essential oils of grapefruit, orange, rosewood, geranium, lavender and thyme give the cream its soothing fragrance.

**Comments:** 'Ten out of ten. Very effective in protecting from sun and elements; went on with no rubbing, comfy on skin – no stinging or tingling, very moisturising' • 'even my husband was happy to wear this because it absorbs so quickly and smells very nicely herbal' • 'goes on better than my usual – expensive – sun prep and makes skin really velvety' • 'hate sun-tan lotions – greasy and terrible smell – but very happy to slap this on, like top-quality body lotion'.

## Malibu Dry Oil Spray SPF15, £2.99/200ml
*Beauty Steal*
**Score: 7.87/10**

Malibu recommend spritzing skin with this fast-drying, waterproof, non-greasy oil 30 minutes before heading for the sun. With a chemical UVA/UVB screen, it can be sprayed through the hair to protect the scalp. Good for men, who tend not to like rubbing sun cream into hairy chests.

**Comments:** 'I was expecting it to be greasy, oily and sticky: it soaked in almost immediately – I am a total convert' • 'as effective as more expensive sun preps; feel texture wouldn't block pores so may help my sun allergy' • 'smells of sun-drenched beaches and piña colada' • 'this

was moisturising but sank in immediately; no rubbing needed' • 'no redness or burning'.

## Estée Lauder Sun Care Body Shimmer Sunscreen, £18/150ml
**Score: 7.77/10**

This moisturising, soothing SPF15 product with a chemical UVA/UVB barrier delivers an instant, gleaming bronze tint and glow. Water-resistant and oil-free, it also contains antioxidant vitamins E and C, plus a 'moisture-locking' lipid complex. Lauder promise a soothing action from the blend of rosemary, peony and sweet violet extracts.

**Comments:** 'Fantastic idea, great product! What pale people have been waiting for: maximum protection and you don't have to keep topping up the fake tan' • 'smoothed into skin easily, without any rubbing; very effective at moisturising' • 'really impressive product: skin looked healthy, divine lounging-on-beach-at-Cannes scent' • 'most of all I loved that little extra sheen on my skin'.

## Liz Earle Naturally Active Sun Shade™ Body Protector SPF15, £17/200ml
**Score: 7.55/10**

This is the highest-scoring of the more natural sunblocks our testers tried: it's formulated without chemical sunscreens, which can trigger allergic reactions in the sensitive-skinned. It includes potent antioxidants from natural source vitamin E, pomegranate and green tea, and has a physical (ie, chemical-free) UVA/UVB barrier.

**Comments:** 'Skin felt wonderfully silky; perfect for using on the face too' • 'really loved this product – it was very moisturising and I didn't burn' • 'luxurious and very good to my skin' • 'I like a physical sunscreen – better than overloading my skin with lots of chemicals' • 'protected my fair skin all day, left skin soft and moisturised'.

# after-suns

Whether your tan lasts or not is down to two factors: how gradually you build it, and the effectiveness of your after-sun. As with sun protection products, these are tricky to test because testers experienced different levels of sun exposure. So we asked them primarily to assess moisturising powers, bliss factor, fragrance – and how soft skin was after use

## Soltan 12-Hour Moisturising After Sun Lotion, £3.99/200ml

**Score: 8.42/10**

This cooling lotion from Boots' admirably affordable own-label suncare is formulated to moisturise continuously for 12 hours, with skin-quenching cocoa butter and soothing allantoin.

**Comments:** 'Light lotion, with very fresh, cooling scent; like a gift from the gods, because I was burnt a couple of days before and it cooled immediately and calmed redness' • 'not as sticky as many creams, easy to rub in and was absorbed totally' • 'a great all-over body lotion' • 'liked the easy fliptop lid' • 'brilliant value'.

## Biotherm Sunfitness Soothing Rehydrating Milk After-Sun, £16/200ml

**Score: 8.16/10**

Biotherm says this smooth, oil-free lotion is suitable for all skintypes except sensitive; rich in shea butter, apricot stone and blackcurrant seed, it's boosted by thermal plankton extract, plus a

compound of six skin-strengthening minerals. NB: it contains 'tan maximiser', aka fake tanner.

**Comments:** 'This was lovely straight from the fridge; skin felt soft and scented' • 'nice citrus smell, cooling sensation' • 'no self-tanning smell, creamy moisturising texture, and was absorbed very quickly' • 'self-tan element gives healthy glow while sun tan developing' • colour is just the best – love this brand!'

## Liz Earle Naturally Active Sun Shade Botanical Aftersun Gel, £12/200ml

**Score: 7.87/10**

A light, cooling gel packed with generous levels of antioxidant green tea, pomegranate and natural source vitamin E, to fight free radical damage, which – like all of the Liz Earle suncare range – is subtly fragranced with lavender.

**Comments:** 'Soothed tight hot skin immediately; incredibly hydrating – skin felt dewy, smooth, moisturised but not sticky; gorgeous smell, too' • 'this was absolutely fabulous: instant relief from sunburn' • 'absorbed very quickly; liked the transparent panel so you could see what was left' • 'sensual, especially when applied by husband'.

## Clarins After Sun Moisturiser Ultra-Hydrating, £16/200ml
Score: 7.83/10

This skin-quenching formula, based on aloe, shea butter, walnut extract, rosemary, camomile and linden, can be used on face and body to help safeguard skin against free radical damage, while prolonging a natural tan. Number one in Clarins' after-sun 'wardrobe'.

**Comments:** 'Gorgeous summery scent: moisture replenishing and skin soothing' • 'burnt area smoother, less tight, and redness faded more quickly than usual • 'quickly absorbed, with no sticky or greasy residue' • 'luxurious, refreshing on sunburned skin' • 'left skin smooth and hydrated'.

## Estée Lauder Sun Performance After Sun Continuous Moisture Cream for Body, £18/200ml
Score: 7.81/10

This aloe-vera-rich greaseless cream claims to boost moisture levels so skin is comfortable and refreshed, while preventing peeling and flaking; antioxidants help minimise cell damage.

**Comments:** 'This was absorbed straight away – my skin felt so soft immediately. Slight sunburn started to go brown by the next day; no sticky feel, and it really prolonged my tan' • 'left a nice sheen on the skin – and I liked the delicate smell' • 'good functional squeezy tube'.

## ❁ ❁ Green People After Sun Lotion, £9.99/200ml
Score: 7.55/10

Post-sun slathering should use up lashings of lotion or cream, so if you're concerned about minimising exposure to synthetic chemicals, this one is the top-scoring, all-natural choice: a skin-cooling, subtly mint-scented lotion, packed with organic aloe vera and calendula. Green People say that it also makes a great everyday body lotion.

**Comments:** 'Lovely and cooling, very easy to smooth in, no dragging and absorbed quickly' • 'tingly, minty, cooling on skin; organic ingredients are a bonus' • 'skin felt cooler and redness went down until skin heated up again, but could just reapply until no more soaked in; relieved tightness'.

WE LOVE...

It may be beauty heresy, but Jo uses organic extra virgin olive oil on her skin when she's been in the sun – packed with antioxidants, and ultra-nourishing. (Gets on your clothes, though, unless you're very careful.) Sarah doesn't burn but moisturises lavishly, post-sun.

111

# spf15 moisturisers

Skin experts insist we should always wear a minimum of SPF15. The easiest way? A sink-in-swiftly moisturiser that creates the perfect 'canvas' for make-up *and* provides an invisible shield against sun damage. It's not just UVB rays that harm skin, but also UVA rays, which do long-term damage – drying and ageing skin, causing wrinkles and potentially leading to skin cancer. Of the winning SPF15s here, several do offer protection against both UVA and UVB, as we detail

*tip* If you're unsure about your current moisturiser, look for the words 'broad spectrum' or 'UVA protection' on the packaging.

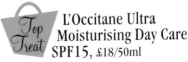

### L'Occitane Ultra Moisturising Day Care SPF15, £18/50ml
*Top Treat*

**Score: 8.6/10**

L'Occitane recommend this for sensitive skins, both normal-to-dry and combination. Very dry-complexioned testers like it too. With vitamin A, sunflower oil and shea butter, it protects against UVA and UVB rays with a physical barrier (titanium dioxide) and two chemicals (cinnamic acid from shea butter and benzophenone).

**Comments:** 'Lovely nourishing cream, totally absorbed to give good base for make-up' • 'skin felt hydrated; good firm texture – make-up went on well' • 'excellent for cold winter days as well as summer' • 'lovely to apply; left my skin very soft'.

### Clarins Hydration-Plus Moisture Lotion SPF15, £22/50ml

**Score: 8.56/10**

Clarins's bestselling suits-all-skintypes moisturiser is, they say, immediately hydrating, and actually increases the skin's ability to retain moisture. With a physical UVA/UVB barrier – titanium dioxide – it includes Clarins's own 'Anti-Pollution' complex, to neutralise the effects of city living.

**Comments:** 'A classic product and a brilliant moisturiser' • 'featherweight – you don't feel it's there' • 'makes you feel a million dollars – I like the pump dispenser, too' • 'at last – a non-oily SPF lotion for my face' • 'make-up went on really well within minutes'.

## Dermalogica Sheer Moisture
### SPF15, £21.60/44ml
Score: 8.3/10

This untinted oil-free moisturiser – see the tinted version on page 130 – offers UVA/UVB protection, with physical (zinc oxide) and chemical (octinoxate) sunscreens, plus plant-derived antioxidants and proteins from walnut seed and olive extracts to protect against pollution and repair skin damage. Testers with troubled skins reported significant improvements.

**Comments:** 'I have the oiliest skin ever, and this absorbed instantly, leaving my skin non-greasy, soft and radiant' • 'after two hours' sun, I didn't change colour or go freckly; it also protected my face from reddening in the wind' • 'not a single breakout with my troubled maturing skin for a month; skin texture looks better and pores smaller' • 'I've not had one rosacea flare-up and my spots are practically nonexistent!'

## Eve Lom Moisturiser
### + SPF15, £38/50ml
Score: 8.3/10

A new creation from superfacialist Eve Lom, this contains extracts of antioxidant red, green and white tea, with chestnut and rosemary. There's a touch of skin-brightening lactic acid, together with soothing bisabolol and yarrow, plus skin-conditioning beeswax and shea butter. The physical sun barrier (zinc oxide plus an extract of edelweiss) protects again UVB but hasn't yet been tested against UVA.

**Comments:** 'This went on like a dream – skin definitely softer and lines less deep' • 'after the initial rubbing in, it dried to a matt-ish finish with a slight sheen' • 'I loved its whipped-soufflé texture' • 'absorbed quickly, and provided a good base for make-up' • 'my skin felt smooth, silky and very soft' • 'lovely simple, classy,

lightweight packaging' • 'after just one use my parched, pinched skin felt more pliable, comfortable, and had a healthy glow'.

## Origins Out Smart Daily SPF25 Naturally Protective Sunscreen, £14.50/50ml
Score: 7.5/10

Origins' new suits-all-skintypes face protector with SPF25 has natural titanium dioxide (a mined mineral) to protects against UVA/UVB, alongside moisture-boosting seaweed extract and antioxidant vitamin C. We own up: we boobed slightly when testing this new product – not realising it was very subtly tinted – but if you're looking for a more natural face-protector with a tad of skin tone-evening colour, this is a great botanical-rich choice. (For other tinted moisturisers, see pages 130-1).

**Comments:** 'Brilliant product: I can honestly say that my skin is in better condition since I have started using this' • 'absorbed nicely; worked well in scorching Mexican sun' • 'goes a long way' • 'squeezy tube easy to transport' • 'nice light colour, so I could wear it without foundation on some days' • 'I really like the fact that it has mineral, not chemical sunscreen'.

# spf15 lipsticks

In summer, you may remember to apply an SPF15 to your face – but what about your lips? They happen to be perfectly angled to pick up sun damage – so the ultimate summer lipstick choice is one which shields against UV rays, yet looks lipsmackingly pretty

In reality, most lipsticks offer a good level of sun protection, because titanium dioxide, the ingredient that gives them dense colour, is also a great physical – as opposed to chemical – sun block. But for summer, we look for something sheerer – so our ten-strong teams of panellists slicked their way through dozens of specific sun-protective lipsticks; these came up smiling. The mantra? Apply frequently. NB: we asked the brands to supply the lipsticks in suits-all-skin-tones shades.

### Bobbi Brown SPF15 Lip Shine, £13
**Score: 8.94/10**

Choose from seven sheer, shiny shades – our testers wore Naked Pink – which Bobbi suggests applying either straight from the stick, with a lip brush or over another lipstick. As a bonus, it's breath-fresheningly minty, with essence of peppermint oil, and a chemical barrier (octyl methoxycinnimate) to guard against UVB rays.
**Comments:** 'I *loved* this lipstick: the colour is fabulous, just how your lips should look; no nasty

smell or taste – if I could give this product eleven out of ten, I would' • 'I really enjoyed this product: it went on smoothly and the natural colour was perfect for me' • 'lovely, natural colour, with moisture you could feel for hours' • 'bullet-size, so crams into a small bag' • 'shiny but not glossy – looked like you've just licked your lips' • 'very conditioning: no need to use a lip balm'.

### Pixi Sheer Lipstick SPF15, £13
**Score: 8.27/10**

Pixi's lipstick is packed with all sorts of goodies: vitamins B, C and E, soothing castor oil, lustrous candellia wax and moisture-attracting hyaluronic acid, delivering a 'sheer, glossy, barely-there' natural finish, according to Pixi, with lip plumping features, too. Our contented testers trialled 'Jenny', a warm, neutral rose stain, from a choice of seven shades, with a chemical UVA/UVB barrier (oxybenzone).
**Comments:** 'Feels really conditioning, but not at all sticky or gloopy; stayed shiny and glossy, and left a slight pretty stain on the lips' • 'love this shade – pretty and healthy looking on its own; glam for evening with a neutral lipliner' • 'funky

little tube that was easy to chuck in my bag'
• 'stayed put on my lips extremely well – no
noticeable smudging, except for on my
husband's cheek!' • 'easy to apply and
substantially less messy than, say, a Juicy Tube'.

## Chanel Aqualumière Sheer Colour Lipshine SPF15, £14

**Score: 7.95/10**

In that so-sexy Chanel packaging, this
super-comfortable glossy lipstick has a cocktail
of ingredients to leave lips soft and supple,
including shea butter and vitamin E, plus a
'volume booster' for lip-plumping effect and
chemical filters to protect skin against UVA/UVB.
Chanel advise powdering lips before application
for staying power. We tested Bahama, from more
than a dozen shades.

**Comments:** 'Fantastic – very moisturising, very
natural colour and made my lips look really
voluptuous and juicy; lasted well and faded
evenly' • 'perfect for summer colour' • 'it's really
lovely to have just one product that does the lot'
• 'classy packaging, classy product' • 'the feeling
on my lips with this was so heavenly that I just
wanted to keep putting it on'.

## M&S Autograph Sheer Gloss Lipstick, £8.50

**Score: 7.31/10**

The transparent, lightweight texture of these
shiny, moist shades makes it easy to wear
brighter colours which otherwise might be too
strong, promise Marks & Spencer. We played
safe, though, with Natural, which testers loved.
The chemical barriers (octyl methyloxycinnimate
and butylmethoxydibenzoylmethane) protect
against UVA and UVB.

**Comments:** 'I loved this lipstick: moisturising, an
SPF, and the shade was perfect – a nude to suit

all skin tones!' • 'such a nice texture, it gives me
a lot of pleasure' • 'great daytime lipstick: lovely
and creamy, stays on for hours – I only needed to
touch up once a day at work – and it left my lips
in great condition' • 'good-looking packaging'.

## ☀ Aveda Lip Tint SPF15, £10

**Score: 7.06/10**

This teeny swivel-up tube of tinted botanical
conditioner has a physical UVA/UVB barrier
(mineral-derived titanium dioxide) along with a
patented moisture complex to protect and
condition that includes organically grown berries,
plus antioxidant algae extract, avocado and
mango butter, and jojoba oil. Oils of wintergreen,
orange and spearmint give the product a
refreshing zing. We tested Copper, from the
range of seven shades available.

**Comments:** 'Gorgeous lipstick – not my normal
colour at all, but so flattering that I will buy it from
now on' • 'very handy beauty product, easy to
apply, lovely colour, softened my lips and the
added benefit of an SPF' • 'ideal summer lipstick,
good for holidays to apply poolside' • 'my lips are
usually quite lined, but this product seems to
have changed the texture'.

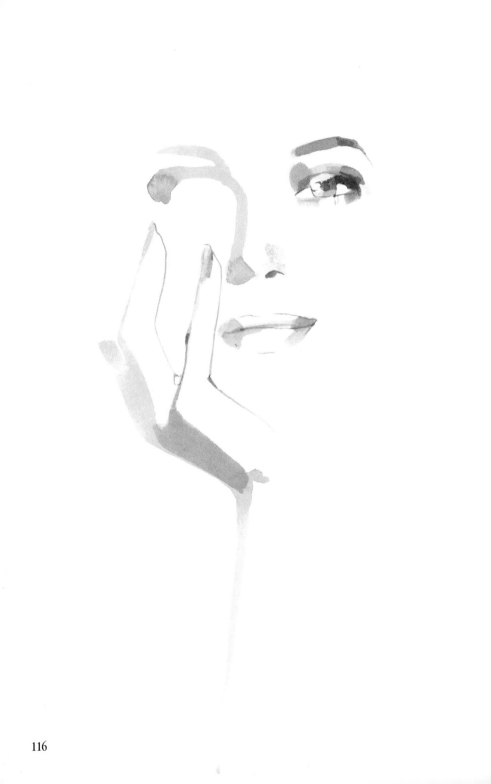

# Skin

In our opinion, there's no greater confidence booster than clear, glowing, radiant skin – at any age. So from everyday cleansers and toners to turn-back-the-clock miracle creams, here are the lotions, potions and creams that truly deliver

# suits -all-skintypes

While there are plenty of cleansers out there targeted at individual skintypes, we were looking for versions that effectively sweep away make-up and grime, whether you're oily, dry, sensitive – or perhaps a combo of all three. For this book, we road-tested another huge new crop of recently launched cleansers, but the originals which impressed our panellists for *The 21st Century Beauty Bible* hardback edition, three years ago, still (clean) sweep the board

## *Beauty Steal* Liz Earle Naturally Active Cleanse & Polish Hot Cloth Cleanser, £10.50/100ml

**Score: 9.5/10**

This is the highest-scoring product we've ever had, in all our years of testing: one woman gave it 11 marks out of ten. From a beauty journalist turned skincare guru, this creamy cleanser is used with hot water and its own muslin cloth (which also works as an exfoliator, hence the word 'polish'). Our testers universally loved the fragrance, which comes from pure essential oils of rosemary, camomile and eucalyptus, which are in there alongside cocoa butter and almond milk. We awarded it our 'Beauty Steal' trophy because, while not a bargain basement outlay initially, it lasts for months and months.

**Comments:** 'Skin felt really clean and fresh after use and very soft' • 'left skin feeling velvety and radiant; texture just right – felt rich on skin' • *'loved* this product! Amazing difference on greasy chin, with noticeably closed pores' • 'took off full "Saturday night make-up" easily' • 'the muslin cloth was strangely satisfying: good to see all the muck that came off my skin' • 'very uplifting fragrance'.

## Eve Lom Cleanser, £42/100ml

**Score: 8.75/10**

Our old friend Eve Lom – one of the world's leading facialists – quite simply changed how we women clean our faces. She pioneered the concept of the muslin washcloth for removing make-up – as opposed to throwaway cotton

> *tip* We've said it before and we'll say it again: the most effective way to remove any kind of cleanser is to use a washcloth or muslin cloth wrung out in hot water and swept over your face. Finish with a cold splash. End of story.

# cleansers

wool – which lightly buffs away dead skin cells and decongests the face. Eve says this solid, aromatic balm is actually four products in one – it's an eye make-up remover, toner and exfoliator as well.

**Comments:** 'I was sceptical at first but after massaging my face, as instructed, all the make-up came off brilliantly' • 'this is the business; great for skin that needs a zing' • 'skin moisturised and *incredibly* soft' • 'feels like you're giving yourself a real facial, not just cleansing'.

## Elizabeth Arden Deep Cleansing Lotion, £14/200ml
**Score: 8.5/10**

According to Arden, this combines the effectiveness of a cream with the lightness of a lotion and leaves the skin feeling smooth and refreshed, removing make-up without stripping the skin of moisture. Here's our testers' verdict.

**Comments:** 'At 2am I wanted something quick and easy to use, and this was it!' • 'just what I expect a cleanser to do: it smelled lovely, removed all make-up and left skin feeling smooth and comfortable' • 'pump-action dispenser ensures no spillage or overuse of product' • 'rich cleanser, absorbed easily, but also easy to rinse off'.

## ✿ ✿ Dr Hauschka Cleansing Milk, £18/150ml
**Score: 8.4/10**

The ingredients in this gentle cleanser are grown organically and biodynamically (in rhythm with the phases of the moon); they include fennel

Sarah's choice is quite simple: Liz Earle's Cleanse & Polish (opposite), which consistently keeps her touchy skin happy and clean. As a long-term fan of solid 'balm-style' cleansers, Jo usually has several on the go: among her favourites are ESPA Gentle Cleansing Balm, £40/60g – 'I love the rose geranium scent' – Green People Organic Femme Cleanser, £17.95/50ml, and a fabulous prototype made up for her by facialist Vaishaly Patel, when she was testing her new signature range. (Watch this space!) NB: two good things about balm-style cleansers – a little goes a long way, and they don't need preservatives to keep them fresh.

extract, jojoba oil, sweet almond oil and clay, with fermented grains ('to assist in breaking down the impurities in the skin', so the Austrian-based all-natural brand tells us.)

**Comments:** 'Silky lotion was easily applied and melted off make-up leaving parched, irritated winter skin hydrated, fresh and comfortable' • 'cleansed effectively – gentle but thorough; left the skin very moisturised' • 'delicious product, more like a treatment than a cleanser' • 'this went into my skin easily and left it feeling very nice – soft, moisturised and fresh'.

# cleansing wipes

Your mother was right when she told you not to fall into bed with your make-up on. But research shows that only 66 per cent of women use a cleanser, so, if you're among the other 34 per cent, this new high-tech generation of cleansing wipes may help to solve the problem

*tip* **This might sound like basic common sense, but the reason a packet of cleansing wipes stops being effective is that women forget to re-seal it properly, so the liquids evaporate. Make sure it's sealed and the wipes stay fresh and efficient, down to the last one.**

Our personal advice, though? Wipes are better for beauty emergencies, or travelling, than as part of your regular regime – for which we'd steer you towards our suits-all-skintypes cleansers, on pages 118-9. Although you'll find three 'Beauty Steals' here, they're probably less economical than regular cleansers – and, as throwaway items, less kind to the planet. Several testers with sensitive skins reacted to some products, presumably because of an ingredient, or possibly the rough texture.

*Beauty Steal* **Nivea Visage Refreshing Facial Cleansing Wipes,** £4.49/25 wipes

**Score: 8.2/10**

Targeted at normal and combination skins, these feature a soap-free emollient plus sea minerals and Pro-Vitamin B5. Tiny 'micro-sponges' take up of gunk and grime, and most testers loved the traditional Nivea fragrance. Dry and sensitive skins should use their Gentle Facial Cleansing Wipes.

**Comments:** 'Extremely easy to use – ideal for daily use and compact enough for travelling' • 'a few wipes removed mascara miraculously; does exactly what it says – convenient, effective, removing make-up and toning all in one' • 'it was wonderful to freshen up with this on a sticky day' • 'particularly soft around eyes' • 'less "wet" than most wipes, but efficient, and not at all drying'.

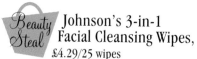 Johnson's 3-in-1 Facial Cleansing Wipes, £4.29/25 wipes

**Score: 8.13/10**

Just nudged into second place by Nivea, these very soft, moist wipes are designed to have the same 'pH', or acid/alkaline balance, as skin, so they shouldn't – in theory – leave your face dry, tight or irritated. They are gentle enough, too, Johnson's claim, for use on eye make-up – even waterproof mascara.

**Comments:** 'Skin was clean and felt better than when I cleanse and tone normally' • 'this really did remove all make-up, cleanse and tone skin and leave it slightly moisturised, with just a few wipes' • 'my teenage son loved these and they cleared my blemishes, except for blackheads'.

Beauty Steal St Ives Energizing Facial Wipes, £3.99/32 wipes

**Score: 7.9/10**

These cleansing tissues say they combine cleanser, toner and moisturiser in a true 'one-stop product' to suit all skintypes. They feature sunflower and camomile extracts and have also done well in magazine awards in Britain.

**Comments:** 'Loved this for cleansing – it didn't fully remove eye make-up, but kept my skin clean and fresh through the day' • 'had a pleasant baby smell; I didn't feel I was cutting corners' • 'this is a fantastic, quick, all-in-one remover, especially if you are feeling tired' • 'snap-shut top is excellent for stopping wipes drying out'.

Beauty Steal Botanics Quick Fix Wipes, £2.99/30 wipes

**Score: 7.7/10**

With soothing mallow extract to calm skin plus other plant ingredients, as the name suggests these wipes marry botanicals from sustainable

## WE LOVE...

Actually, we don't love. Frankly, we've never found any cleansing wipe we really like, and even when we're too tired to think, we somehow go through our regular cleansing ritual. But then we are beauty eds who practise what we preach. So we bow to our testers' opinions on this one.

sources with high-tech and are suitable for sensitive skins, say Boots.

**Comments:** 'Very efficient, packaging good and nice fragrance: I'd use these again' • 'my skin felt very clean but quite dry' • 'easy to carry around' • 'removed eye make-up very well' • 'excellent – large wipe left skin comfortable and clean'.

## Estée Lauder Take It Away Longwear Makeup Remover Towelettes, £16/45 wipes

**Score: 7.66/10**

A definite 'beauty splurge' compared to the other winners, but testers appreciated the stay-moist packaging, fresh fragrance and gentle-on-the-skin, good-size cloths. Super-saturated with a cleansing emulsion that hydrates and softens, they also include the skin-conditioning amino acid arginine.

**Comments:** 'I'm addicted! Skin feels fresh and comfortable, very easy to use, don't dry out, ideal for travelling, freshening up at work, or lazy moments' • 'very soft cloth, no dragging; removes even waterproof mascaras' • 'nice light fragrance' • 'no need to rub at make-up – just lifted it off'.

# skin toners

Toners are way down on our own beauty must list, as we explain below, but some women love them, so our panels of ten testers tried literally dozens, including several natural and nearly natural options, which scored very highly

Personally, we believe that a toner is an entirely optional step in a beauty regime: a great cleanser will do all that's needed to get skin perfectly clean. So we rarely use them: a splash of cold water leaves our skin feeling invigorated and sparkling. But if you do want the fresh feeling a toner delivers, make it really gentle. Harsh toners can actually upset your skin's acid (pH) balance and/or over-strip skin, sending oil glands into overdrive; all the beauty experts we respect suggest that an alcohol-free version is best for all skintypes – so that's what we tested. (When left to its own devices, skin is clever enough to rebalance itself: even oily skins tend to become less oily if a gentler toner is used.)

## Liz Earle Naturally Active Instant Boost Skin Tonic, £8.95/200ml

**Score: 8.66/10**

This good-value, fresh-smelling, alcohol- and astringent-free toner contains natural ingredients including aloe vera, cucumber and vitamin E plus essential oils. Every one of the testers commented on the delightful fragrance (could they please have a scent with the same bouquet, they pleaded), and it scored ten out of ten with several, making it far and away the highest-scoring toner.

**Comments:** 'Skin felt sparkly clean, refreshed and hydrated' • 'my face looked softer and skintone brighter' • 'loved the gorgeous uplifting smell' • 'my skin positively glowed – pores seemed minimised without skin feeling tight; it's so delicious I'm recommending it to all my friends' • 'packaging was clean and pleasing' • 'does exactly what it says on the bottle – revitalises, soothes and tones for instant radiance'.

### *Beauty Steal* ✳ ✳ Neal's Yard Rosewater, £4.55/100ml
**Score: 7.88/10**

Made from pure rose absolute, this fragrant, 100 per cent natural toner helps to cool, balance and soothe all skintypes without drying. Rosewater has, of course, been used for centuries by great beauties seeking gorgeous skin – and it's as effective today as it was back in the Middle Ages!

**Comments:** 'This was a fantastic toner that made my skin feel wonderful – not tight at all' • 'also felt lovely on cotton wool pads spread over my eyes' • 'helped to cleanse my skin completely' • 'I really loved the beautiful old-fashioned smell of roses; I used the toner by sprinkling a few drops on my hands, then pressing into my skin' • 'it was really good for refreshing tired eyes and face; my skin looked cleaner and the pores were definitely reduced' • 'my boyfriend is also a fan and now uses this every day in secret'.

### Decléor Tonifying Lotion, £15.50/250ml
**Score: 7.72/10**

This light pink alcohol-free toner has essential oils of lavender and petitgrain, with orange, kiwi, mallow and lime blossom waters. Most testers said their skin felt 'toned', but some said they thought it felt tight.

**Comments:** 'Skin looked fresh, unclogged, smooth and radiant' • 'removed all the final traces of cleanser' • 'made my skin feel smooth and pampered' • 'a good toner if you are a heavy make-up user – skin felt refreshed and hydrated' • 'smells heavenly' • 'skin felt and looked very clean after use' • 'my moisturiser sank in beautifully and I was able to apply make-up straight afterwards'.

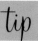 **tip** If you're looking for a toner and you can't tell from the label whether it's alcohol-free, use your nose. If there's skin-stripping alcohol in the formulation, you can literally smell it, in a nasal whoosh. Another clue is to look for the word 'gentle' somewhere in the name, which usually means no alcohol. As our testers observed with every product, the fragrance of a toner is key to its pleasure factor; quite simply, you have to love the scent to love using the toner – so follow your nose.

### Lancôme Tonique Douceur, £16/200ml
**Score: 7.15/10**

A true beauty classic – Jo's Mum was using it 30 years ago! – this is described lyrically by Lancôme as 'soft and fresh as morning dew' – and our testers certainly found it to be refreshing and revitalising. Several commented favourably on the fact that it was straightforward to get exactly the right amount of product out through the hole in the top, without getting it everywhere.

**Comments:** 'After using this toner, my usual moisturiser seemed to sink in deeper, so my lines were plumped and hardly noticeable' • 'this definitely gave my skin a little extra moisture boost' • 'leaves the skin very fresh and hydrated, and made me feel very clean' • 'I really liked the product's wonderful smell of Parma violets and roses'.

# facial oils

Slurp, slurp, slurp. That's the sound of a thirsty complexion drinking in a facial oil packed with goodness. French beauties swear by them; now, facial oils are catching on outside La France – and these, our panels of ten testers declared, are the true wonder-workers

Don't look for a 'beauty steal' here, because facial oils are pricy: they're pure raw ingredients, with no water or petrochemicals. But you only need a very few drops and they are often far more economical than the price tag suggests. As wannabe-natural beauties, we love facial oils because they are – mostly – free of preservatives: germs don't breed in oil, so the makers don't need to add extra chemicals. Tip: keep facial oils out of daylight – unless they're in dark glass bottles – as light will diminish their power.

## WE LOVE…

Jo loves facial oils, and massages in a couple of favourites on alternate nights: one that was blended for her personally by facialist Vaishaly Patel, and Daniele Ryman Seeds Oils Anti-Ageing Serum, £17/30ml, exclusive to Boots, 'which leaves my skin truly glowing'. Sarah's favourite is Aromatherapy Associates Renew Rose & Frankincense Facial Oil (see opposite for details and description of what it suits).

### Top Treat Circaroma Skin Gentle Facial Serum Rose Otto + Apricot, £25/28ml

**Score: 8.22/10**

This radiance-boosting facial oil really impressed our testers. Virtually all its ingredients are organic, and with softening apricot oil and rose otto, this will restore balance to parched and delicate skin, Circaroma promise.

**Comments:** 'I was sure my skin would erupt in spots but it looks clearer, brighter, smoother – and stubborn spot marks are healing' • 'I felt this regulated my skin's own oil production' • 'fine lines on the brow and eye area were smoothed out' • 'people said I looked radiant' • 'skin softer, plumper, springy to touch' • 'reduced redness on cheeks and nose after three weeks'.

## ✸ Clarins Skin Repair Beauty Concentrate, £31.50/15ml
**Score: 8.21/10**

Clarins say this 'SOS' for skins should be used nightly for sensitive complexions, or as needed on skins that have 'flared up'. It includes soothing liquorice extract, soya and avocado oils plus essential oils of lavender, mint and marjoram.

**Comments:** 'A miracle: my skin's looking smoother, clearer, and younger' • 'skin looks and feels peachy' • immediately softer' • 'used it on a burnt hand: two weeks later hardly any scarring'.

## ✸ Clarins Huile Santal Facial Oil, £26/40ml
**Score: 7.88/10**

A second Clarins winner, this time a classic packed with sandalwood oil and lavender, and perfect, they say, for skins that are dry or have high colouring.

**Comments:** 'Absolutely brill! Immediate improvement in softness and radiance' • 'a godsend for dry skin after a new baby' • 'no dryness, skin feels wonderful, make-up sits better and hasn't settled into fine lines; very economical' • 'forehead lines are softer and acne scars on cheeks have faded substantially'.

## ✸ ✸ Aromatherapy Associates Renew Rose & Frankincense Facial Oil, £27/15ml
**Score: 7.5/10**

Intended for dry, more mature complexions and tired skin which may be losing its firmness, this anti-ager blends rose and frankincense in a base of vitamin E-rich peach kernel and borage oils.

**Comments:** 'Fantastic – skin is soft, smooth, fresh, glowing' • 'love the smell: beautiful to use' • 'really helped during a cold when my skin was badly dehydrated' • 'has really made a difference to fine lines' • 'after a while, skin looked plumper'.

## ✸ ✸ Decléor Aromessence Neroli, £25/15ml
**Score: 7.5/10**

Aromessences are the cornerstone of Decléor's range, to be used individually or as a 'booster' for other skincare. The Neroli Aromessence – based on orange blossom – is designed for all skintypes, and should sink in swiftly.

**Comments:** 'Skin was smoother, more radiant, nourished and moisturised, very good around eyes and other dry areas; seems to help fine lines too' • 'colleagues asked what I've been using to keep my skin looking good in the cold; I would recommend this to everyone' • 'dry spots and unevenness in tone gone, and skin looks rested'.

# moisturisers

Mostly, we think, all skin needs to look peachy is a good, long drink of moisture, not necessarily with turn-back-the-clock ingredients or other frills. Our panels of devoted beauty hounds reported to us on dozens and dozens of moisturisers to help you take a short cut to those that simply get on and do the job

We assembled our teams carefully so that testers were assigned moisturisers that suited their complexions: light lotions or creams for normal-to-oily, richer formulations for thirsty ones. And if you like your creams to be packed with plant ingredients, rather than petroleum-derived ones, you'll be pleased to know that several of the products featured in this section are packed with skin-quenching botanicals.

### Estée Lauder Hydra-Complete Multi-Level Moisture System, £21/30ml
**Score: 8.6/10**

'Your skin's not ageing – it's thirsty' is the slogan for this super-high-tech cream, which was inspired by studies of climate change in the controlled environment of the Biosphere centre, in Tucson! Lauder claim this cream helps insulate skin against harsh climatic changes in day-to-day life, thanks to a formulation including aloe butter, hyaluronic acid, 'mineral-rich biowater' and Indian kokum butter. Our combination-skinned testers

were assigned the appropriate cream for their skintype, but there's one for dry skins, too.

**Comments:** 'Sank in instantly and skin was silky and soft, looked really fresh and fine lines were reduced; like the velvety texture that melts into skin; after three weeks my complexion looks really radiant' • 'skin much plumper within an hour' • 'perfect consistency, smells like fresh linen, lots of people have commented on how good my skin looks – it glows!' • 'provides a lovely smooth base for make-up; after a few weeks, the lines round the top of my cheeks are much smoother; I would buy it' • 'within 24 hours my face was softer, smoother, plumper' • 'a lifesaver after having my baby; moisture perfectly balanced and fresh again, instead of tired and drained'.

### Liz Earle Skin Repair Light, £12.50/50ml
**Score: 8.56/10**

We tested so many moisturisers for this category that any brand which earned a place in the ranking deserves praise – but Liz Earle has two winners (see the second, opposite). Skin Repair Light is the new, super-light version created for normal/oily/problem skin, in a pump dispenser. Key ingredients, as with the original, are echinacea, avocado oil and natural-source vitamin E.

**Comments:** 'Lovely product – have just ordered more so I'm never without; perfect for oily skin owing to its lightness; the natural products seem to soothe and tame skin even in hard water areas' • 'skin was immediately brighter and felt lighter and less product-y than usual' • 'very light and easy to spread; provides a slightly dewy look; skin feels able to breath' • 'like the clean pleasant smell and silky rich creamy texture' • 'sinks in very quickly, perfect under make-up, even eye shadow' • 'skin definitely looks better after using this product' • 'I'm a Liz-oholic and this was wonderful; make-up stayed on longer and looked smoother; made me look radiant' • 'easy and pleasant to use, and it worked! Highly recommended'.

## Lancôme Aqua-Fusion Oil-Free Fresh Gel Cream, £25/50ml
**Score: 8.3/10**

Lancôme's bumph for this product virtually requires a PhD in chemistry to decipher, but in brief: it's based on a special water enriched with 16 elements, from manganese to sugars, which is said to deliver time-released moisture over 24 hours. Our normal-skinned testers used the gel-cream; there's also a fluid for combination skins and a rich cream version for thirsty ones, all infused with a 'summer garden fragrance'.

**Comments:** 'Skin texture was softer, smoother and brighter; loved the fresh smell; good base for make-up' • 'skin was almost velvety, instantly – it even looked a little brighter' • 'after a month my skin is in really great condition, even though my diet has been a bit hit and miss, which usually makes my skin look dull and lacklustre' • 'sinks in straight away; foundation seemed to glide on and blend in much more easily; make-up stayed put

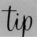

**tip** Central heating literally sucks the moisture out of skin, so if you switch it on for the colder season, do keep an eye – or a fingertip – on your skin and switch to a more nourishing cream for a few months if it becomes drier. NB: rooms with plants in, or simply bowls of water, have naturally higher moisture levels.

longer, too' • 'I normally think people are lying when they say a moisturiser makes them look instantly better but that is really the case – made skin velvety-soft and gave it a healthy glow; after a month, it looks brighter and clearer than for ages; also you only need a tiny amount'.

## ※ Liz Earle Skin Repair, £12.50/50ml
**Score: 8/10**

One of Liz Earle's early signature products, this has now sold over a million jars. 'An ideal base for make-up' (they promise), it's also a sinks-in-fast night treatment, with generous levels of botanicals including skin-saving echinacea, EFA-rich borage oil, vitamin E, avocado oil, natural beta-carotene and hop extract. It comes in two formulations– as well as Skin Repair Light – our testers reported on the dry/sensitive version, but there's one for normal/combi skin, too.

**Comments:** 'Ten out of ten: made skin look radiant and healthy; Liz Earle is a goddess and should be given the Nobel Prize for Services to Skincare' • 'really moisturising – great for my dry skin; made it very smooth and soft' • 'loved the smell – a fresh summer day' • 'perfect make-up base' • 'this is how all moisturisers should be: my skin is in heaven – smooth, clear and clean looking; I'm very happy!' • 'you only need a little bit'.

## Kiehl's Ultra Facial Moisturiser, £12/50ml

**Score: 7.94/10**

A light, moisturising cream from the 'cult' beauty brand which L'Oréal snapped up, a few years back, this is fragrance free, colorant free and contains a significant amount of squalene, Kiehl's tell us – an ingredient derived from olives which closely resembles the skin's natural sebum. It's appropriate for combination skins and comes in a stylish plastic bottle that's great for travelling. Testers were divided about the smell.

**Comments:** 'Surface of skin was smoother, almost matt in a pale, translucent way; my husband – unusually – said my skin looked "lovely and smooth" when I only had this and no make-up on' • 'skin seemed to glow, but wasn't shiny' • 'suited my 30-year-old daughter's combination skin very well and made it feel silky' • 'loved this; felt like a lovely light lotion but gave me all the moisturisation I look for in a face cream – leaves skin looking and feeling really smooth and soft; plumps up fine lines; small bottle but lasted ages' • 'skin looks less crêpey, plumper, seems thicker' • 'think it tightened the pores slightly' • 'very good base for make-up'.

## Clinique Superdefense Triple Action Moisturiser, £22/30ml

**Score: 7.4/10**

Oops: since it has an SPF25 and UVA filters, we should probably have tested Superdefense in our SPF15 moisturiser category. Notwithstanding that boob – inevitable when you're sending out over 13,000 products! – this new moisturiser packs powerful antioxidants into a mega-moisturising cream, available in three formulas for different skintypes: Normal to Dry, which our testers trialled, Normal to Oily and Very Dry. Each, of course, is fragrance free, allergy tested – and, Clinique tell us, non-acnegenic, so shouldn't cause spots.

**Comments:** 'I was delighted: my skin looked smoother and felt softer, balanced and healthy; lovely base for make-up, soft and receptive to foundation, a clean slate and non-greasy, so make-up doesn't slide off' • 'you don't need to use a huge amount as it's so creamy' • 'I have less spots and dry patches; skin feels like it is being fed – I just love the texture' • 'unscented, so fantastic for sensitive skins and non-greasy, so I might even go without foundation' • 'I'd definitely buy – even without checking the price' • 'no other moisturiser has cleared up both my spots and dry patches; I feel so much better about my skin'.

## Nuxe Crème Fraîche, £19.50/60ml

**Score: 7.4/10**

Subtitled 'Energizing Emulsion', the French cult brand Nuxe calls this 'a feast for your skin': light yet creamy, and based on what Nuxe describe as 'eight vegetal milks', or plant-derived milky-looking juices obtained by macerating seeds, flowers or fruits in water and oil – in this case from lupin, white pea, almond, coconut, soya and oat.

**Comments:** 'Noticed an immediate softness and dewiness to my skin and was particularly pleased about the hydration, which made it plump without being greasy; very fresh natural smell' • 'gives a plumped dewiness to skin, making it look really fresh and alive' • 'sank in very quickly, leaving a dewy surface just right for make-up or to go bareface with a touch of blusher' • 'skin looked more fresh, plumped and healthy with more luminosity and more youthful looking' • 'very rich and moisturising, but sinks in very well; excellent base for make-up – foundation went on evenly after only one minute' • 'lovely luxurious moisturiser'.

## ✻ ✻ Neal's Yard Rose & Mallow Moisturiser, £10.50/40g

**Score: 7.35/10**

If you like your creams as pure as possible, this is our highest-scoring all-natural moisturiser – touted by Neal's Yard as a 'must-have winter skin saver' for its richness. Healing almond oil, nourishing mallow and rose essential oil – which targets redness and broken capillaries – feature high on the ingredients list, with an extra splash of rosiness from rose absolute.

**Comments:** 'Skin was immediately softer, smoother and looked brighter; dry and oily patches evened out' • 'very rich texture, smells divinely of roses' • 'skin felt and looked brighter and smoother without feeling like I've piled on the anti-ageing products' • 'good for days and nights when tired and skin needs a quick boost, feels luxurious' • 'I also use it on décolletage and ears' • 'skin seemed more hydrated and bright, with a degree of radiance; also felt smoother and tighter; over weeks had a firming effect' • 'seemed to protect my skin in cold weather'.

## ✻ Dr. Baumann Intensive Normal and Mixed, £35.10/30ml

**Score: 7.3/10**

Another botanically rich product, from a small German company with a growing fan base which is committed to animal welfare and to minimal packaging. It features vitamins E, D, shea butter and jojoba oil, and comes in a version for Normal and Mixed skins (our testers' allocation), and Dry.

**Comments:** 'No-nonsense product that reminds me of a tub of ointment; thick, white, unscented cream – velvety texture glides on to the face, leaving skin feeling soft, looking fresh and radiant; make-up glides on easily' • 'skin looked brighter immediately; at a ball people kept commenting how well I looked – fresh and bright – despite

having two young kids' • 'got me through a nasty cold, face moisturised without the usual dry cold-y flakiness' • 'very rich creamy texture, but sank in fairly quickly, considering; people say my skin looks in good condition' • 'skin was less shiny most of the time; kept it evenly moisturised; also kept spots at bay, and a couple of pigmentation patches under each eye have faded' • 'didn't like this product initially because of the texture, but have changed my mind completely because of the results after a few weeks'.

**WE LOVE…**

An all-natural cream from Germany – Lavera Laveré Hydro-Sensation Energy Cream, £23.40/50ml – has been Jo's unswerving number-one moisturiser choice since she discovered it at a German natural products show a few years back – and she's delighted it's now available here, as it suits her very sensitive skin perfectly. Sarah loves the Lavera product, too, but for her dry skin her mantra is simple: 'Moisturise thoroughly, then do it again.' She loves Aromatherapy Associates Renew Triple Rose Moisturiser, £40/50ml, thrust into her paw by make-up artist Jenny Jordan, who says it's a miracle – and it is! Especially preceded by Renew Intensive Skin Rose Serum, £26/50ml; when your skin smells heavenly.

# tinted moisturisers

The perfect tinted moisturiser evens out skintone and gives a hint of healthy glow – without making you look like you've drifted off the set of *Footballers' Wives*. Our quest for sheer, clear, complexion-perking coverage involved testing dozens of tinted moisturisers on our panels of ten, who declared these the winners

*Top Treat*

## Stila Sheer Colour Tinted Moisturiser SPF15, £20/50ml

**Score: 9/10**

We weren't surprised to find this is one of Stila founder and make-up artist Jeanine Lobell's all-time favourites: our testers were blown away by its blendability and evenness of finish. With an SPF15, it's said to be ideal for normal-to-dry skins – although, Stila insist, 'it won't add any unnecessary oil to oily skins'.

**Comments:** 'I don't usually use tinted moisturiser but this one was perfect, adding a sheer sheen to my skin' • 'loved this – I had a cold and in consequence was looking very pale and pasty, but this made me appear instantly healthy again' • 'lovely natural look – perfect for daywear' • 'gives effective moisturisation without being greasy; covers imperfections and lasts for up to eight hours'.

## Dermalogica Sheer Tint Moisture SPF15, £21.60/44ml

**Score: 8.88/10**

You want oil-free hydration, a full-spectrum SPF15 sunscreen – which protects from ageing UVA rays – and a sheer wash of colour? Well, that's what Dermalogica promise with this lightweight cream, which uses natural earth minerals (iron oxide) rather than synthetic colourings. It's also rich in plant-derived antioxidants from walnut seed and olive fruit extract – said to provide the highest level of protection of any natural antioxidant.

**Comments:** 'Extremely easy to apply; smooth, with good coverage' • 'where has this been all my life? I've never used tinted moisturiser before and now I'm a convert' • 'fantastic if you just want to even out skintone'.

## Yves Saint Laurent Teint de Jour Tinted Matt Moisturiser, £22/40ml
### Score: 8.33

For a matt effect rather than dewiness, this is a great choice, with bamboo powder to absorb oil and leave skin shine-free for 'at least eight hours', they swear. According to YSL, Teint de Jour also helps fight fatigue 'with an active biological ingredient that helps re-stimulate cellular metabolism' – and, notwithstanding its matt effect, it increases skin moisture, too.

**Comments:** 'Went on smoothly with no tide marks – excellent' • 'I didn't feel like I had anything on, but had a healthy natural glow' • 'at long last, a tinted moisturiser that does its job perfectly' • 'pleasant, fresh-floral scent; skin still velvety at the end of the day'.

## Laura Mercier Tinted Moisturiser, £30/44ml
### Score: 8.22/10

Why didn't anyone think of this before? Make-up genius Laura Mercier cleverly offers her tinted moisturiser – which also has a higher-than-average SPF20 – in a choice of six shades. Laura's tip? 'Use foundation during the week, and tinted moisturiser on weekends.'

**Comments:** 'Skin looked healthy – good coverage for my acne-prone complexion, which has some scarring' • '*loved* this – has better coverage than my usual SPF, so can replace this and remove the need for foundation' • 'very comfortable'.

 **tip** Goofed with your self-tanner? That's where tinted moisturisers come into their own as a quick fix: apply them to the white 'striped' bits and your tan will be instantly evened out. Or, better still, mix half and half with self-tanner, and blend, very carefully, into the paler areas. You can use a synthetic foundation brush to apply this mix, for accuracy. And, if you're putting product on pale skin, do remember: it's tinted, so don't stop at your chin.

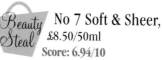 ## No 7 Soft & Sheer, £8.50/50ml
### Score: 6.94/10

From their recently-revamped range, this is No 7's won't-break-the-bank replacement for Illuminating Tinted Moisturiser – which featured in our last book. It's a sheer wash of colour, featuring an SPF15, with moisturisers that go on working for 12 hours and light-diffusing particles to leave skin looking radiant.

**Comments:** 'This is very nice and light to use for the summer months; easy to blend' • 'although it didn't disguise blemishes – which, admittedly, I wouldn't expect a tinted moisturiser to do – this product did manage to even out my skintone' • 'I thought it was scarily dark at first, but it blended well and was great for creating a glow effect – gave a really attractive sheen to my skin' • 'helped to disguise my thread veins'.

# anti-ageing eye treatments

The eye zone is the first area to show up signs of ageing – and for a lot of women, laugh lines aren't that funny. So – hallelujah – even our most cynical testers were impressed by some of the turn-back-the-clock eye treatments that are now available

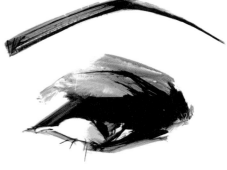

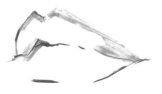

You'll notice that several of the winning products incorporate a 'hot' new technology, said to 'prevent the micro-contractions responsible for wrinkle formation' – in other words, Botox without the Botox, using compounds that are deliberately given high-tech, medical-sounding names. Frankly, we're pretty sceptical that any cosmetic can rival line-zapping treatments from a cosmetic dermatologist (though we'd still rather you didn't have those!), but it's undeniable that our panellists – who tested these creams over several months on one eye only, monitoring the ongoing results – were won over by these winners. With all but a few products, the instant results were far outweighed by the evident benefits after six weeks and more.

 ### Guerlain Issima Success Eye Tech, £55/15ml
Score: 8.27/10

Guerlain say this is a double-whammy product, not only targeting fine lines and wrinkles but also sagging of the fragile eye contour area – and promise that from the first application, the upper eyelid looks tighter. With an outstanding score from panellists, this fragrance-free formulation contains 'Injectine' – who thinks up these names? – to improve absorption of vitamin C, magnesium aspartate, tormentil, and 'blue gold', 'an alloy of pure gold and an extract of abyssal algae', a signature ingredient of the Issima range, which may explain the hefty price tag.

**Comments:** 'This actually works; lines were smoother and finer, eyes a little brighter, slight puffiness much reduced; excellent at hydrating, and a slight difference in crêpiness – my husband thought I looked less tired and friends believed I'd had several early nights!'
• 'I wear glasses and have never kept up eye treatments before, but this cream is so good: after six weeks, fine lines disappeared, I had a more "wide eyed" look, puffiness was reduced, wrinkles less prominent' • 'this sank straight into the skin beautifully' • 'gorgeous packaging and I would definitely buy the product' • 'people commented the skin around my eyes was line-free'.

### Crème de la Mer Eye Balm, £85/15ml
Score: 8.05/10

Our second-highest scorer was also a seriously blow-the-budget choice, from the 'cult' Crème de la Mer range. In addition to the famous marine 'broth' found in every Crème product, this soothing formulation incorporates Brazilian malachite, an illuminating mineral that diffuses redness and creates the optical illusion of blurring lines.

**Comments:** 'This has an amazing consistency – glides easily over the skin, sinks in quickly, not greasy, but you can feel the moisture there hours later' • 'there was some instant improvement – skin seems more elastic and softer round whole eye area; this is a good base for eye make-up; after six weeks, fine lines and wrinkles are less obvious' • 'this is an expensive purchase, but a jar a lasts a long, long time'.

## Estée Lauder Advanced Night Repair for Eyes, £30/15ml
Score: 7.77/10

Lauder's Advanced Night Repair is a true 'beauty classic', one of the first to incorporate high doses of antioxidants, and this is its night-time eye-treatment cousin, designed to rebuild the barrier of the super-thin skin around the eyes, also targeting puffiness and dark circles. Active ingredients include extracts from yeast, white birch, mushroom, algae – and that antioxidant complex of mulberry, saxifrage, grape and skullcap.

**Comments:** 'Definitely improved bagginess after six weeks, wrinkles less prominent, lines smoother and finer, some improvement in dark circles and crêpiness' • 'did not irritate eyes' • 'fine lines definitely blurred, touch of crêpiness disappeared – I've found my miracle eye cream and will be buying this for ever' • 'I noticed a difference within a week and so did other people; fine lines definitely went in under six weeks, and whole eye area was brighter and "lifted"'.

## Vichy Myokine Corrective Anti-Wrinkle Peri-Ocular Care, £14.50/15ml
Score: 7.66/10

In this non-greasy, hypo-allergenic gel/cream from Vichy – who are part of L'Oréal, where technologies are often shared between brands including Vichy, Lancôme and L'Oréal Paris (see below) – the supposedly muscle-inhibiting ingredient is called 'Adenoxine™', derived from magnesium and adenosine, plus cafeinine (vitamin C and caffeine). Almost a 'Beauty Steal'.

**Comments:** 'Wonderful: immediate softening of harsher lines, and finer lines less obvious; over time fine lines definitely reduced in depth, became softer and less noticeable; skin elasticity improved, and it looked fresher' • 'had an instant lifting effect' • 'velvety smooth product that's moisturising and soothing, absorbed really well and left no greasy residue, so make-up didn't slide' • 'really do think it reduced some fine lines after six weeks; also slight improvement in brightness, dark circles less noticeable'.

## L'Oréal Wrinkle De-Crease Eyes, £12.99/15ml
Score: 7.65/10

An affordable eye treatment that also claims to tackle the problem of fine lines through another patented ingredient – theirs is called Boswelox™ – which minimises those wrinkle-causing mini-movements. Here's what our testers thought…

**Comments:** 'Light yet effective, absorbs easily and quickly, light pleasant fragrance, after six weeks: fine lines seemed to disappear, wrinkles less prominent, eye area lifted, dark circles reduced, and I got compliments from friends' • 'within days, there was a noticeable improvement in lines' • 'put this on husband's deep lines and wrinkles too – we have a baby and our eyes show how exhausted we are – this was a miracle worker' • 'reduced puffiness in the mornings, and dark circles; skin a bit tighter round eye area' • 'fabulous for contact lens wearers'.

### ✳ Aveda Tourmaline Charged Eye Cream, £25/50ml
**Score: 7.5/10**

Fine-powdered tourmaline helps 'bounce' light off the skin in Aveda's Tourmaline range – which also scored well in Skin Brighteners, on page 25 – making lines less obvious. Alongside this mineral ingredient you'll find Indian pennywort, lycopene – a potent antioxidant – moisturising glycerine and hyaluronic acid, beta-carotene, cooling cucumber and light-diffusing silica, to brighten dark circles.

**Comments:** 'Good packaging and pointed nozzle tip: silky, matt-finish cream glided on with no greasy film, though very moisturising' • 'this made a very good base for eye make-up, and I noticed an immediate brightening effect – my skin was fresher and smoother' • 'after sustained use, dark circles not so dark; I hadn't used

**The best anti-ager of all for eyes?** A pair of big, wide-armed, 'Jackie O' sunglasses, which shield the vulnerable eye zone from UV damage.

concealer recently and I had no noticeable circles – eye area looked fresh and healthy' • 'after six weeks, huge dramatic effect on crêpiness, fine lines seemed to disappear, wrinkles less prominent, skin smoother and finer, eyes brighter'.

### Lancôme Resolution Yeux, £32/15ml
**Score: 7.5/10**

This third winning offering from the L'Oréal stable – a thick cream that needs warming before applying with fingertip – also contains an ingredient designed to 'reduce dermo-contractions'; this time, they've called it D-Contraxol™.

**Comments:** 'After six weeks, fine lines less pronounced, wrinkles less prominent, skin smoother and finer and crêpiness reduced' • 'some instant blurring of fine lines, and all-round improvement after six weeks – very good product' • 'no instant improvement until I put on foundation, when I seemed to have a fresher appearance round eyes' • 'slight but wonderful improvement in dark circles: definitely freshened eye area, foundation glides on better and stays on: very impressed and think this is a good investment' • 'skin felt beautifully moisturised: a good maintenance product'.

# miracle creams

The question we're asked by everyone, everywhere we go, and all the time, is, 'Do miracle creams really work?' And we can put our hands on our hearts and say, 'Yes, some really can help turn back the clock'

We admit it: despite sitting through endless skincare launches where we're force-fed cosmetic science – some of it cod – we started out pretty cynical about miracle creams...until we started our *Beauty Bible* series of books in 1996. Still, we thought, we'd better test them, by sending each of them – as with every product in the book – to ten appropriately aged women, for their opinions. Our challenge: use the cream/lotion/serum on one side of your face, monitor any improvements – by comparing with the non-treated side – and report back, after a few months. Each time we write a new book, we test all the new creams – and we've long since lost count of the number of testers who've e-mailed us after a few weeks to ask if they can start using their anti-ageing potion on both sides, because the difference was starting to become so apparent. So our verdict – based on what hundreds of women have told us – is that when it comes to wrinkles, there really is such a thing as a miracle. And it needn't break the bank.

 *Beauty Steal*

## Time Delay Rejuvenating Day Cream SPF8, £9/50ml
(exclusive to Boots)

**Score: 8.71/10**

In their wisdom, just as our last book, *The 21st Century Beauty Bible*, was published, Boots renamed this product as above – it was previously called Time Delay Repair Face & Neck. Aside from that – and subtly tweaking the fragrance – they reassure us that the highly effective formulation has not been changed. A no-nonsense cream at a truly outstanding price, this came in well ahead of the competition – and none of the creams we've tested since has outperformed it. It can be used on face and neck, and active ingredients include pro-retinol and a 'pro-lift' complex from white lupin extract, together with powerful antioxidants. There is a moderate SPF8 in there – fine for winter, but not for summer, we'd advise.

**Comments:** 'I thought age-delaying creams were a con – but this one has changed my mind' • 'I looked glowing – and was even asked if I was pregnant, several times, because of it!' • 'marked reduction in fine lines; my partner made nice comments' • 'totally transformed my skin's appearance – my face looks years younger than I am, and I'm 100 per cent sold on this' • 'my skin felt plumper, younger and looked fresher; loved this – it looks and feels expensive' • 'a few people mentioned how well I was looking' • 'definite improvement in tone'.

## Estée Lauder Re-Nutriv Ultimate Lifting Creme, £150/50ml

**Score: 8.4/10**

Ritzily packaged and with a sky-high price tag, this is truly in the realms of skin luxuries – a Mercedes-Benz of an anti-ageing cream, with active turn-back-the-clock ingredients that include green tea and resveratrol – from grapes – white birch extracts and creatine, an amino acid. Most of our testers concurred that the only downside to this cream is the cost.

**Comments:** 'This cream is definitely a miracle cream – it changed my skin from dry to glowing and although I didn't have deep lines, my fine lines have almost gone' • 'definite improvements in skintone and texture – this really is a gorgeous cream to use' • 'reduction in lines on neck, bright radiant glow to skin; my open pores are also diminished. Lovely to use'.

## Elemis Pro-Collagen Marine Cream, £75/50ml

**Score: 8.4/10**

This was the first serious anti-ageing cream from the respected 'spa' brand, incorporating ginkgo biloba, to boost circulation, seaweed extracts – the 'marine' element – and absolutes of rose and mimosa, combined together in a nourishing base that includes carrot seed extract, jojoba oil and shea butter.

**Comments:** 'This really is a miracle cream – and a little goes a long way, so, although it's expensive, it should last a long time' • 'people at

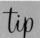 **tip** Our biggest anti-ageing secret is yoga (although there was precious little time to practise while writing this book). It oxygenates skin like no cream ever can, melts away frown-lines, generally de-stresses and, we feel, makes you feel better about the whole ageing process. We think it should be on the NHS and plan to go on doing it till we're 100. Enough sleep and lots of still water – eight large glasses at least, daily, between meals – are completely vital too.

work – men – seem to be giving me a second look and I feel much more confident after using it; – I've seen a dramatic improvement' • 'I was very sceptical that any product claiming to reduce lines/wrinkles would work, but I've been proved wrong. I'm hooked' • 'this will be on my Christmas list as a special treat' • please send me a bucketful of this cream'.

## Elemis Liquid Radiance Cell Renewal System, £65/2 x 10ml

**Score: 8.35/10**

Elemis's latest anti-ageing innovation enters the ranking just a teensy bit behind Pro-Collagen Marine Cream: they call it a 'skin detox', which helps to neutralise the damaging effects of free radicals, packing a mega-dose of no less than 15 antioxidants, plus other vitamins. A two-phase treatment programme, it's not designed to be used all the time but for 30 days in all, whenever the complexion needs a boost – making it, promise Elemis, 'more luminous and satin-like, while reducing pore size'.

**Comments:** 'Ten out of ten: before my skin was grey and dull – now even my husband commented on how my skin glowed and was fantastically bright, very soft, with a great reduction in fine lines; I can't praise this product enough' • 'skin definitely looks younger' • 'divine smell, very lightweight, instantly absorbed milky lotion; after first week, skin definitely clearer, softer and pores refined, more even toned – amazing!'

## *Beauty Steal* Almay Kinetin Daily Moisture Cream SPF15, £18.95/40ml

**Score: 8.28/10**

A rich, nourishing formula which was the first to use kinetin – an anti-ageing ingredient now turning up in quite a few skincare products, and which was formerly available by prescription only from dermatologists – Kinetin's a highly stable antioxidant from green, leafy plants. The cream is 100 per cent fragrance free and allergy tested – Almay are famous for that – and additionally features an SPF15. With just one exception, our testers were wowed.

**Comments:** 'I'm addicted – fabulous! Gives that "I've just had a facial feeling" – soft and smooth to the touch, perfectly moisturised' • 'this made a significant difference – lines were minimised, especially round the eyes and mouth' • 'after eight weeks' use, this melted years off my face' • 'I'm overjoyed – my skin is smoother, looks younger, glows, and elasticity has been restored; my boyfriend and Mum have both noticed a difference' • 'this is brilliant to use under make-up' • 'my skin looks brighter, fresher, slightly younger; fine lines have been improved, and there's some improvement on my forehead furrow'.

## Philosophy When Hope Is Not Enough Serum, £28/29.6ml

**Score: 8.2/10**

The 'sister' product to the original Hope In A Jar (opposite), this scored even higher marks with the ten women who trialled it. A light, fluid gel, it can be worn under moisturiser on drier skin, and harnesses amino peptide technology with a large dollop of skin-brightening vitamin C. None of our testers had a negative word to say about this.

**Comments:** 'Lives up to its promise – quite noticeable reduction in bigger grooves and wrinkles, as well as a moderate improvement in crêpiness' • 'brilliant stuff – my skin looks like I've had a facelift and several people have said that I'm looking well' • 'made my skin look like I live on a healthy diet of fruit and water – and I couldn't stop touching its baby-softness' • 'it took about two weeks to see the difference but it was worth the wait – I didn't even feel the need to wear make-up some days' • 'I love the pipette-style dispenser – very scientific, yet the smell is very holistic, herbal, floral and natural' • 'also claims to retard hair growth, which, amazingly, appeared true – upper hair regrowth on my top lip slowed down'.

## Caudalie Vinosource Riche, £23/40ml

**Score: 8.16/10**

Caudalie products were originally formulated to take advantage of the highly potent antioxidant grape by-products of the vineyard owned by founder Mathilde Thomas's parents, near Bordeaux. This features stabilised grapeseed polyphenols – more powerful than vitamins C and E – as well as chestnut extract and omega fatty acids, and is specifically designed to ultra-moisturise very dry skins.

**Comments:** 'Smooth creamy texture, smells fresh and sinks in very nicely; lovely feel, and skin instantly more hydrated' • 'after several weeks; skin smoother and definitely plumper, much brighter and fresher, more alive-looking, lines round eyes filled out – moderate improvement in bigger wrinkles' • 'compliments include one person asked if I'd had a facelift' • 'vast improvement on throat area crêpiness; I feel better in me' • 'best new product I've tried in ages; feels lovely and does what it promises – a small tube goes a long way'.

## Philosophy Hope In A Jar, £30/56.7g
### Score: 8.14/10

This cream is a favourite with celebrities, make-up artists and cosmetic surgeons, available in versions for normal-to-dry skin, which we tested, and combination. Despite the tongue-in-cheek name, it was originally created for the medical market, and contains beta-glucan, a powerful antioxidant.

**Comments:** 'Fantastic – beautiful texture, and my skin is younger, brighter, firmer and more radiant' • 'I've sensitive skin and this is the first product I've had no reaction to – silky, luxurious, a real treat to use' • 'skin brighter, almost glowing, with an improvement in fine lines – I loved this' • 'fine lines have reduced over 12 weeks – difficult not to use it on the left side; it will have some catching up to do!' • 'lasts ages, with the most wonderful velvet texture – skin' is 100 per cent brighter' • 'people are commenting that I look younger; my husband can see a difference too'.

## ☀ Origins Make A Difference, £26.50/50ml
### Score: 7.85/10

This was the highest-scoring of the more natural ranges we tested – and to be honest, we're only awarding it the daisy for naturalness because none of the other botanical offerings came

anywhere close to delivering similar anti-ageing benefits. File under 'more natural' than 'natural', then: a lightweight cream-gel in which active ingredients include algae, a corn-derived sugar and rose of Jericho, a plant known for its ability to withstand almost total dehydration.

**Comments:** 'This really is a miracle cream – by far the best moisturiser I've ever used, delivering excellent results; colleagues have commented how well I look' • 'I've really enjoyed using this – the smell and texture are gorgeous; worth sticking with it, as the results just keep getting better' • 'I look less tired' • 'skin is brighter – I just look more healthy' • 'I really loved this delicious product and will buy more when it runs out'.

# neck creams

A good neck cream works wonders, instantly plumping and smoothing. But some have real long-term effects, too – as our testers found, after applying twice daily over two months. For this new book, our teams tried another round of neck creams but none of them scored higher than the original – and impressive – winners in *The 21st Century Beauty Bible*

## WE LOVE...

Sarah has always been fanatical about moisturising her neck and décolletage. She uses mainly Estée Lauder's Daywear Plus Moisturiser SPF15, £26/50ml and Liz Earle's Naturally Active Skin Repair Moisturiser (opposite). Jo makes her own neck cream, the recipe for which features in her book *The Ultimate Natural Beauty Book* (also published by Kyle Cathie, £14.99).

*Top Treat*

### Clarins Extra-Firming Neck Cream, £34/50ml
Score: 9.19/10

Active ingredients in this very high-scoring cream include ginseng, mallow extract and moisturising honey, plus antioxidant vitamin E and rice extracts. For optimum results, Clarins recommend exfoliating the neck once a week to remove any dead cells: for great scrubs, see pages 166-7, or use a muslin cloth – or even a flannel.

**Comments:** 'Increasing improvement, especially in crêpey skin at the middle and front of the neck' • 'under my chin is firmer and less saggy' • 'neck looks loads younger and smoother' • 'loose skin tighter and less lined' • 'the bit under my jawline and chin is firmer, more defined' • 'delicious smell – a little goes a long way' • 'lines on my neck had disappeared by the end of the two month trial'.

### Chanel Ultra Correction Anti-Wrinkle Restructuring Lotion, £58/50ml
Score: 9/10

Light and non-oily, this lotion boasts an SPF10 – good news for necks, which are so vulnerable to sun damage. It's designed to work on dark spots and wrinkles, incorporating liquorice (to regulate hyperpigmentation), emollient canola oil and shea butter, a vitamin E derivative, and what Chanel call a 'Life Cycle Regenerator'. Chanel prescribe a ritual massage to enhance the benefits of this cream, which our testers diligently followed.

**Comments:** 'My neck has lost its greyness and is not so crêpey-looking' • 'rich texture, smelled like heaven: massaging the skin makes me aware how much better it seems – the best cream I've ever used' • 'my dermatologist said my skin was very moist and smoother than usual • 'skin looks plump, well-fed – "lifted" '.

## *Beauty Steal* ☀ Liz Earle Naturally Active Skin Repair Moisturiser, £12.50/50ml

**Score: 7.85/10**

With the usual high level of active botanicals you'd expect from Liz Earle, this is also our 'best budget' recommendation. It's actually a facial nourisher, but they were so confident of its performance as a neck cream they submitted it for this category – and our testers loved it. Active natural ingredients include echinacea, borage oil, avocado, beta-carotene, hop extract and wheatgerm.

**Comments:** 'My neck, which tends to be crêpey, is smooth and soft – a significant difference' • 'smells divine, nice creamy texture – left skin smoother and soft' • 'I'm raving about this – it actually does more than it says on the jar!' • 'cleavage in Christmas party frock – achieved with a Wonderbra – wasn't as crêpey' • 'my neck looked less like plucked chicken skin – skin had a lovely sheen and healthy glow'.

## ☀ ☀ Jurlique Neck Serum, £50/30ml

**Score: 7.55/10**

This sinks-in-fast, lightweight gel is 100 per cent natural, with high quantities of organic ingredients, and Jurlique (one of our favourite natural companies) promise us that the soya on which it's based is not genetically engineered. Botanical actives include frankincense and myrrh, ginkgo flavonoids, vitamin C and oils of jojoba, rosehip, avocado and evening primrose.

**Comments:** 'My neck looks slightly younger, smoother, more hydrated and clearer' • 'definitely less crêpiness after just two weeks' • 'sinks in fast; lovely fresh and natural smell – lines are less visible' • 'skin on neck and décolletage noticeably smoother' • 'I'm amazed how much smoother my skin feels – definite improvement in fine lines'.

# line-smoothers

This is a new category of products that we predict is going to be huge: perfect for the Botox-phobic, these line 'fillers' can be dabbed and smoothed into wrinkles to make them disappear. But do they really work? Read what our testers have to say

Though she doesn't often use the products featured on these pages herself – she's usually in too much of a hurry! – Jo has given both the La Prairie and Prescriptives products as gifts to friends, who tell her they now can't live without them. Sarah uses both products (not together) when she's filling stressy and her forehead furrows are more than usually, um, furrowed; but, for eye lines, just dotting on more moisturiser (as in our tip, opposite) does the trick.

When Jo demonstrated the winning product in this category on a TV breakfast show a while back – on a willing fiftysomething guinea pig who professed herself totally blown away by the results – the station's switchboard collapsed under the weight of calls, and supplies of this 'Polyfilla for wrinkles' had to be airlifted from all over Europe and even the States to cope with demand. But these are definitely products where practice makes perfect: it's important to experiment with different techniques to see whether the line-filler is best used under make-up or applied on top of foundation/powder for a more flawless appearance. We've found they are most effective over moisturiser – under foundation – gently tapped into areas of deeper wrinkles, such as frown- and laugh-lines.

Neither of the two products featured here scored a high average mark, mainly because even though older ones gave them top marks, younger testers 'couldn't see the point' – they wouldn't, would they? – which brought the average down.

We do think they are worth trying as a 'quick fix' alternative, before you book in for expensive collagen/filler/Botox jabs, of which we are decidedly not fans. Line-smoothers are based mostly on silicone, which is entirely harmless when applied on top of the skin.

## Prescriptives Magic Invisible Line Smoother, £27/15ml

**Score: 6.93/10**

Prescriptives describe this as 'an intuitive gel', which fills in lines and deep wrinkles to re-create a supple, even surface. It's packed with optical diffusers which 'bounce' light off skin, and soften any unevenness. Several of our testers opted to use this as an all-over-face primer – which is an expensive method – but they loved the results!

**Comments:** 'Ten out of ten! Beautifully silky and soft, perfect for under eye area; skin looked younger and clearer; most lines disappeared; make-up went on well after' • 'my mother, who is 50, loved it – made a big difference to her; she went out and bought it immediately' • 'perfect after a late night to perk up eye area – made skin look brighter and younger' • 'no stinging and felt very light on the skin' • 'invisible under foundation but skin felt a lot smoother and fine lines less noticeable' • 'never felt skin or eye area so soft and silky' • 'very easy to apply with fingertips; lines seemed to blur and soften' • 'make-up sat on it perfectly' • 'only needed a tiny bit and one friend commented how flawless my skin looked'.

## La Prairie Rose Illusion Line Filler, £65/30ml

**Score: 6.9/10**

This is a skin treatment as well as an instant fix: alongside the silicone, light-deflecting polymers and optical diffusers, La Prairie have incorporated moisturising glycerine, marine collagen, vitamin E and their own exclusive Cellular Complex. And there's a bonus: the rose scent of this product wafts

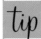

**tip** Dry-looking skin always appears more lined, so to blur the appearance of lines instantly, take a tiny dab of moisturiser on the tip of your finger and tap it into the area: skin looks immediately 'dewier' and less lined.

blissfully up the nostrils, as some testers commented. Again some testers just couldn't resist using this as a primer.

**Comments:** 'The lines under my eyes and on my forehead seemed blurred; overall tone of my skin was firmer and plumper, skin appear more flawless and glowing; texture improved' • 'people said that I glowed; someone said my skin looked very peaches and cream' • 'you need less than the size of your little finger nail' • 'fine lines didn't disappear, but did look less obvious'• 'better than the primers and flash balms I've used in the past; it lifted my whole face' • 'I'm totally positive about this product; my skin felt springy, wrinkles seemed less prominent, lines were definitely smoother and finer, and it lifted the area: was told several times how well I looked' • 'I used this on one side of my face, which looked brighter and less tired – radiant' • 'my skin just got better during the day – more refined and glowing' • 'this was fantastic as a primer – my foundation just glided on, and it helped my eye make-up; you only need a tiny amount'.

# facial exfoliators

Dingy skin can be brightened by using scrubs and exfoliators. The ideal scrub is gentle to skin, leaving it vibrant – not angry and red. Our teams of 'scrubbers' tried literally dozens, each for a month. Here are the ones that impressed them – including several natural options

W e're sceptical about the current craze for home dermabrasion kits and micro-peels, so we decided not to test them. There's a risk that women will think 'more is more' – and strip away layers of skin that are vital protection against UV and pollution damage. These scrubs and exfoliants are kinder options which should be absolutely fine for all but the most delicate English-rose complexions.

## WE ♥ LOVE...

We've long used muslin cloths and hot water for facial exfoliation. Recently, though, we've tried **Origins Modern Friction** (right) and **Liz Earle Naturally Active Gentle Face Exfoliator** (opposite) to great, skin-brightening effect – and with no reactions from our notoriously touchy skins.

 *Top Treat* **Guinot Gommage Biologique Gentle Face Exfoliator,** £23.25/50ml

Score: 8.5/10

We actually tested this scrub for our previous book in the 'Instant Face Savers' category – but because it's an exfoliant, we felt it was more at home here, despite its instant face-saving action. It's the enzymes in the formulation that provide the exfoliating action, softening the links between cells before they're sloughed away. Gommage Biologique also includes green tea extract and shea butter and, say Guinot, is good even for sensitive skins.

**Comments:** 'Skin much improved – sort of "plumped-up" '; loved this' • 'I looked all rosy and attractively flushed; it's great that it works so fast – really, a super-quick boost' • 'my face felt fresh for most of the day' • 'I felt as if I'd had a facial – but without the expense' • 'left me with firmer, brighter, softer skin'.

## Origins Modern Friction, £27.50/125g

Score: 8.4/10

A terrific score for a brand new product that Origins launched specifically as a gentle alternative to microdermabrasion products. This creamy buffing paste is based on a mix of rice starch, skin-brightening scutellaria (skullcap), cooling and soothing cucumber and aloe leaf – lightly fragranced with lemon and bergamot essential oils. Gentle enough to use two or three times weekly – but it will sting if it gets in your eyes.

**Comments:** 'My skin looked brighter, fresher, more even toned and cleaner immediately after, and felt so soft and smooth. After a month, it's wonderful' • 'really does give my skin a more youthful appearance' • 'lathers up well so you don't have to use much' • 'my T-zone isn't so greasy now' • 'has minimised my open pores to a truly astonishing degree'.

## Guerlain Issima Smoothing Exfoliator, £20.50/75ml
**Score: 8.1/10**

A smooth, creamy fluid that 'liberates spherical micro-particles to gently exfoliate deep down' (in Guerlain-speak). Women who react to AHA/fruit acids should be aware there's a fruit acid complex, although Guerlain have also incorporated soothing mallow extract and 'Calmitine-S complex', as they call it.

**Comments:** 'Skin felt refreshed, glowing and really clean – it removed small blemishes without damage and took away the day's lived-in look!' • 'gorgeous smell; comfortable, not abrasive, when rubbed over the skin' • 'foundation went on more easily and smoothly' • 'has converted me to exfoliating to put my skin right after the elements have done their worst'.

## ❋ ❋ Pennyhill Park Jasmine & Frankincense Face Polish, £16/50g
**Score: 8.06/10**

This rich, creamy, blissful smelling exfoliator gets its buffing action from tiny particles of walnut shell

**tip** Before exfoliating, you should always cleanse the skin thoroughly and warm it with a hot flannel to soften dead cells; then use your chosen scrub in ultra-gentle, circular movements. Focus on dry patches, and areas around the nose and the chin 'groove' – few complexions need all-over scrubbing.

and jojoba beads and features high levels of organic ingredients (including carrot oil). It was created for Pennyhill Park's organic day spa by ultra-natural beauty brand Circaroma.

**Comments:** 'I raved about this to my boyfriend and he agreed my skin was really soft and smooth' • 'lovely rosy glow on my cheeks and skin felt brill' • 'nice consistency, easily rinsed off with warm water' • 'smelt gorgeous, really expensive' • 'I'm pleased it's organic – saving the earth while indulging me'.

## ❋ Liz Earle Naturally Active Gentle Face Exfoliator, £10.50/70ml
**Score: 8.05/10**

Another recently unveiled product, blending moisturising cocoa butter with jojoba beads (from jojoba oil), designed to buff without scratching. Eucalyptus gives a refreshing smell and has antiseptic powers.

**Comments:** 'Made my very sensitive and acne-prone skin smooth, calm, clear and glowing; my skin feels definitely much more balanced now' • 'wonderful: my skin feels clean and much softer and looks healthier generally; dry skin, spots and pimples all seem to have lessened' • 'lovely energising smell'.

# face masks

A face mask is a blissful way to wake up a tired face – and the few minutes while it's working its magic can provide welcome 'time out' from a pressured life. So here's our rundown of the masks which revive, replenish and restore skin's vibrancy

## WE LOVE…

Jo usually whips up her own face mask, but when time's short, reaches for Brightening Treatment, £9.25/50ml, from Liz Earle Naturally Active; she adores the camphor smell and the fact it puts back the glow in just two minutes. Another favourite is B Kamins Chemist Bio-Maple Diatomamus Earth Masque, £34/130g, which is miraculously brightening on her Sahara-dry skin. Oh! Jo just stole Sarah's absolute fave: Ben Kaminsky developed this super moisturising skincare for his middle-aged wife and it is genius: not only brightening but also truly plumping for Sarah's thinnish face.

We asked for masks to suit all skintypes, but be aware that some may prove too rich for oily skins. Although we tested literally dozens of new face masks for this book, these classic favourites from our previous rounds of testing are still unrivalled.

### Top Treat Guerlain Invigorating Moisture Mask, £26/75ml
### Score: 9/10

Our testers gave an exceptionally high score to this ultra-nourishing mask, which contains mallow, ginkgo biloba and Guerlain's 'Calmitine-S' complex of soothing, protective active ingredients, which – they tell us – makes this a perfect choice for sensitive skins.

**Comments:** 'Light and silky, with a tea-rose scent, it smoothed and relaxed, plumped, softened and moisturised' • 'so light you didn't realise you had anything on your skin – left a lovely glow, with brilliant brightness' • 'this product is heaven – and made my make-up last longer' • 'skin felt like a baby's bum – soft and supple' • 'can be used instead of moisturiser before applying make-up' • 'felt ten years younger – that's a miracle!'

## Elemis Fruit Active Rejuvenating Face Mask, £21.50/75ml
**Score: 8.55/10**

Elemis warn that a natural tingling sensation is normal with this mask, which should be left on face and neck for 10-15 minutes. Botanical skin brighteners include kiwi and strawberry, while shea butter and macadamia nut oil have a nourishing effect. They claim it's good for smokers, as it enhances circulation.

**Comments:** 'High pamper factor – felt expensive and luxurious' • 'total relaxation; skin didn't need make-up next day and my husband remarked how silky my face felt' • 'utterly rapturous!' • 'great whenever skin is looking tired and dull' • 'gave a lovely "porcelain finish" and a polished gleam' • 'my skin glowed with health and was evenly toned' • 'skin soft and smooth for four days'.

## Sisley Express Flower Gel Mask, £49/60ml
**Score: 8.5/10**

Lily and iris give this a light, flowery smell, while extract of organically grown sesame helps deliver a super-fast moisture boost. Ideal for all skintypes, but especially for tired and dull complexions.

**Comments:** 'Miraculous! My skin looked so good, I abandoned foundation for the evening' • 'love that it needs too be left on only for three minutes' • 'light, refreshing gel with a scent like cut grass' • 'skin was "plumper" for a day or two' • 'gave a healthy glow; clarity immediately enhanced' • 'good before a night out, as skin looks instantly soft'.

## Shiseido Moisture Relaxing Mask, £30/150ml
**Score: 8.44/10**

Shiseido suggest a special massage technique – described on the packaging – to turbocharge the benefits of this moisturising mask, which contains

**tip**  Hands respond in the same way as faces to a good mask, appearing instantly smoother, softer and less dingy. So treat the back of your hands and fingers, as well as your face and neck.

hyaluronic acid, Shiseido's own 'phyto-vitalising factor', glycerine, thyme and tea-rose extracts. According to Shiseido, even stressed skins are left 'feeling as though bathed in cool water'.

**Comments:** 'Results with this were near-magical – skin glowed and looked exceedingly healthy' • 'used over three weeks, the effects were visible – smooth, healthy-looking skin' • 'skin looked rested and alive' • 'this was hydrating, cooling, softening and radiance-boosting' • 'soufflé-like texture – truly a delight to apply'.

## Liz Earle Naturally Active Intensive Nourishing Treatment, £9/50ml, including cloth
**Score: 8.02/10**

Ultra-moisturising ingredients include borage oil, comfrey extract, shea butter, glycerine and St John's wort oil, subtly fragranced with rose geranium essential oil. It comes with one of Liz's signature muslin cloths, the best way to remove any face mask, in our experience.

**Comments:** 'Benefits seemed to last a couple of days – every time I used this, my skin felt like a soft, ripe peach' • 'skin seemed more "plumped up" • 'really relaxing feeling' • 'useful, too, for backs of hands in winter' • 'skin felt calm and relaxed with a blushing bride tone – hooray!' • 'skin looked altogether brighter and pores were tighter'.

# beauty supplements

These take a big investment and a lot of faith, because you won't see any results for months. That puts off lots of women, but – as our testers found – it can be worth persevering, for improvements in skin texture, stronger nails, shinier hair and vitality

## WE ♥ LOVE…

Jo is unswervingly devoted to Imedeen Time Perfection, £37.50 for one month's supply, having over the 12 years of popping Imedeen occasionally had her skin assessed by the high-tech equipment used by Imedeen to assess skin density – and seen with her own eyes that hers is extremely thick and resilient, for her age – which she'd rather not think about! Sarah is also becoming a fan of Imedeen's anti-ageing Expression Line Control skincare range.

We've long been converts to skin supplements, so we were especially fascinated by this trial, which required our *Handbag Beauty Bible* testers to take skin/hair/nail nutritional complexes over a period of at least three months – the minimum time in which you'll see significant results. We've always believed that beauty isn't just about what you put on your skin but how you 'feed' it, so we aren't surprised that many of our testers were pleasantly surprised, too. However, although we sent out a dozen supplements, none earned praise from every single tester. So the relatively low average scores reflect the marks of some testers who raved about them and others who were underwhelmed.

## BioCare Hair & Nail Complex,
£21.85/one month's supply
Score: 7.32/10

From a nutritional supplement company we rate highly, a complex to help maintain healthy hair and nails, combining silica-rich horsetail, lysine, folic acid, pantothenic acid, biotin, copper, zinc, vitamin E and vitamin $B_{12}$. It's recommended that one capsule is taken three times a day, with food.
**Comments:** 'Skin glows more after one month – several people say how well I look and how shiny my hair is; after three months, skin is rosy, glowing, plump and healthy, very soft – most noticeable difference is my nails, stronger, quicker

growing, smoother and shinier; I'll keep taking the pills!' • 'after month two, my hair has a new lease of life, definitely bouncier, more voluminous, easier to style – everyone notices! After three months, definite improvement in skin softness; baby fine hair feels so much thicker; nails growing, too – how I love these pills!' • 'definite improvement in fine lines after month two, hair thicker, nails looking their best ever, fabulous! Loads of comments from men: my skin looks the best it has in years; hair's in great condition – I can't afford not to buy these'.

## Imedeen Prime Renewal,
£49.50/one month's supply
**Score: 7/10**

Imedeen, brand leaders in skin supplements, have recruited the eternally gorgeous Jane Birkin as the 'face' of this supplement (shot by David Bailey). It's designed for post-menopausal skins: as oestrogen levels drop, collagen levels reduce – up to 30 per cent in the first five years after menopause. We selected testers aged 55-plus to trial these tablets, in which Imedeen's signature Biomarine Complex™ is found alongside isoflavones and a new ViTea™ protection complex, based on vitamins C and E, zinc, camomile, white tea, tomato and grapeseed, targeting fine lines, wrinkles, age spots and skin firmness.

**Comments:** 'After two months my hairdresser said hair is less dry and shinier; nails stronger, shinier and growing much quicker – after three months, skin brighter, less crêpey dry, younger looking; really worth taking these' • 'after two months, my daughter said my skin looked fresher; after three my husband noted my skin was better' • 'after one month, eyes and neck less crêpey, skin softer, fine lines round eyes less; improvement continues over three months; neck is much smoother, crow's-feet almost gone, generally skin is improved, nails really better; shall continue'.

**tip** Do read the instructions carefully and follow them, take the supplements consistently and give them time to work. Also, check for contra-indications, particularly if you have an allergy to shellfish or fish, because many contain a fishy ingredient.

## *Beauty Steal* Healthspan Nurture Anti-Ageing Skin Nourishment Supplement,
£7.95/60 capsules (one to two months' supply)
**Score: 7/10**

Healthspan – a mail order vitamin company – formulated these affordable supplements in tandem with Dr David Harris, of The London Clinic of Dermatology, combining Omega-3 oils from fish and borage oil with high-strength antioxidants grapeseed extract, plus vitamins A, C and E. For best results, Healthspan recommend these are taken while using their skincare products, but our testers tried them with their own regimes.

**Comments:** 'This product has made a subtle improvement to my hair, skin and nails; biggest difference is my hair, which has more bounce and falls into a style more easily' • 'took time, but my skin is healthier looking, hair shinier and less flyaway – my hairdresser says the condition is better; also feel better in myself' • 'nails are smoother, far less peeling, not breaking off as easily; much stronger and more flexible at the end of three months; fine lines are better; I've been very surprised and pleased by the results' • 'skin much brighter and more radiant, looks younger; slight improvement in fine lines'.

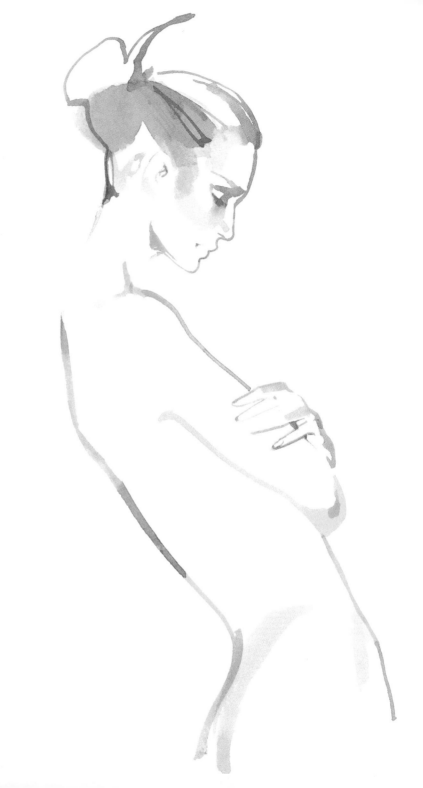

# 7

# Body beautiful

We can't all be born with a
body like Elle Macpherson's –
but we can all make the
most of what we've got.
From cellulite smoothers to
skin silkifiers, hair removers
to super scrubs, we bring
you the best body beautifiers

# body moisturisers

Buying a body lotion that isn't a pleasure to use, and doesn't do the job, triggers a beauty dilemma: do you ditch it – wasteful and expensive – or grin and slather it on until the end of the jar? We suggest, instead, following the recommendations of our panels of slatherers, who declare these the top body treats

Our panels tested literally oceans of recently launched lotions and creams for this category, with some new entries – from Champneys and L'Occitane – earning a place in the ranking for their power to leave skin touch-me silky, smooth and hydrated. The rest are tried-and-tested high performers who've impressed our human guinea pigs in the past – and we'd say they're well worth trying.

including lavender, tea tree and camomile, to soothe, smooth and moisturise. It lived up to all its promises, say our rhapsodic testers, several of whom gave it ten out of ten.
**Comments:** 'Very quickly absorbed, smelt nice, almost like aromatherapy, no greasy residue and softer skin – full marks!' • 'smooth silk texture, heavenly gorgeous smell that really awakened my senses; skin felt nourished and cared for – plus perfect pump-action dispenser' • 'easy to apply – even on slightly hairy legs!' • 'worth the price'.

### Dermalogica Body Hydrating Cream, £19.30/222ml
Score: 9.2/10
Non-greasy and rapidly absorbed, this combines exfoliating alpha-hydroxy acids from sugar cane, apple and milk with essential oils,

### ☀ REN Wild Yam Omega 7 Body Cream, £39/250ml
Score: 9/10
Featuring wild yam – long used for menopausal women – to moisturise and help boost skin lipids, this high-scorer also contains sea buckthorn berry oil, a potent source of

Essential Fatty Acids. Many women like to use a more natural product on their bodies and, while not 100 per cent, this is trying pretty hard. One tester gave it 11 out of ten!

**Comments:** 'Almost instantaneously absorbed, dry areas disappeared and my skin felt as smooth as velvet' • 'my worst areas of dryness – shins and heels – were cleared up; I really enjoyed using this product' • 'light unobtrusive smell, generous-sized pump dispenser; seems to have banished late-winter scaly skin' • 'all my skin was softer – even my husband noticed' • 'I only had one ingrowing hair after waxing, while using this – and normally I have loads' • 'my new best product for my very sensitive skin'.

## Clarins Renew-Plus Body Serum, £31/125ml
Score: 8.89/10

Extremely good results, in a highly competitive category, for this body 'anti-ager', which features high levels of pro-retinol – a form of vitamin A – to enhance cellular renewal, along with gently exfoliating wintergreen, olive, cashew nut oil and Madagascan white lily – which is rich in vitamin C and, so Clarins trumpet, has an exceptional ability to retain water. It's specifically anti-ageing and suitable for anyone of 30-plus, they recommend.

**Comments:** 'Glistening, dewy skin on first application with definite firming action, noticeably on thighs' • 'a week's use of this improved texture, tone, faded stretch marks' • 'body felt fresher, more alive, with thighs better toned after a week of using this perfect-consistency serum' • 'skin felt like velvet and looked more toned and even – definite "pamper-yourself" effect' • 'left an attractive sheen on my skin' • 'a real miracle!'

## Jo Malone Lime Basil & Mandarin Body Lotion, £35/250ml
Score: 8.83/10

From the renowned London facialist whose cult brand was snapped up by the Lauder empire, this moisturising and nourishing lotion is available not just in this zesty scent – one of her bestsellers – but in a wide choice of other Jo Malone signature fragrances.

**Comments:** 'Skin felt moisturised and fragrance lasted well all day' • 'skin very soft and luminous, and a little goes a long way – a real treat' • 'made my dry skin tingle nicely after the shower' • 'skin felt softer and smoother after a week' • 'like putting silk on skin – my whole body felt classy' • 'this immediately quenches dry skin' • 'if I could afford it, I would buy this product by the crate'.

## Decléor Système Corps Moisturizing and Firming Body Emulsion, £24/250ml
Score: 8.66/10

This light, creamy milk is suitable for all skintypes but especially, so Decléor say, for dehydrated, dull skins or those recovering from pregnancy/weight loss or gain – and stress. The moisturising elements include coconut oil, vitamin E and nourishing meadowfoam oil.

**Comments:** 'A great all-round product; super smell, quick and easy when you're rushing in the morning' • 'dry patches were gone from knees and elbows – I loved this' • 'smoothed and pampered, like I had an invisible velvet coating on my skin – a dream!' • 'left slight silky sheen on skin; softer skin on upper arms and fewer skin "blips"' • 'elbows were instantly softened'.

## Olay Total Effects Body Anti-Ageing Moisturising Treatment, £10/150ml

**Score: 8.62/10**

From their mid-priced, turn-back-the-clock range, this stars Olay's unique 'VitaNiacin' ingredient, formulated to combat the 'seven signs of ageing': dryness, roughness, lack of firmness in areas like arms, uneven skintone, dullness, fine lines and wrinkles. In some countries, they offer a money-back guarantee if you're not satisfied. NB: one tester experienced a sensitivity reaction to this cream, so discontinued use.

**Comments:** 'Definite improvement in skin softness in about a week, especially behind knees, and my ankles' • 'from day one, my parched, neglected skin was restored to softness' • 'the best I've tried – after a few days I was happy to show my embarrassing heels in public again' • 'skin looked less dry and wrinkly; crêpiness diminished, flakiness gone' • 'could use this in the morning before getting dressed, as it absorbed quickly; wonderfully light but luscious'.

---

*tip*

Forget everything you ever heard about 'trapping moisture' by applying body lotion when skin's damp – all that happens is that you dilute the lotion or cream you are putting on. Instead, for optimum benefits, massage it into skin that's been patted dry with a towel.

---

 *Beauty Steal*
## Champneys Skin Comforting Creamy Body Butter, £8/375ml

**Score: 8.5/10**

A rich blend of shea, olive, mango and cocoa butters, this intensive nourisher – from a new range available at Sainsbury's, created with lots of input from the therapists at Champneys' spas – has been specially formulated for dry and dehydrated skins. It has added lingonberry oil, rich in soothing and protecting Omega-3 fatty acids, along with a 'mood-balancing' blend of geranium, orange and cedarwood essential oils.

**Comments:** 'Loved the big pot, warm buttery nutty-ish smell and rich, thick luxurious texture; skin was immediately soft and smooth and looked less line-y' • 'smoothed over the skin like silk, sank in incredibly fast and kept me well moisturised; loved the comforting smell; good to use before bed, as the smell lingers and you can still smell it in the morning' • 'wonderfully softening on the skin and lovely fragrance lasted all day' • 'my skin feels fantastic; smooth and silky – even my husband has commented!'

## L'Occitane Almond Milk Concentrate, £28/200ml

**Score: 8.5/10**

With use of this light 'whipped' cream over three to four weeks, L'Occitane promise, after extensive testing, that skin will be firmer and smoother. Our testers were asked to comment only on the product's shorter-term benefits – which are down to the concentration of almond oil and almond milk – but were impressed, nevertheless.

**Comments:** 'My favourite product! Lovely delicate almond smell; made a real difference to the texture of dry and bumpy areas; also a slight improvement in firmness' • 'skin was immediately smooth and soft' • 'truly amazing results after two weeks: I followed the massaging instructions and skin was tightened and toned, as well as being enriched and nourished – the claims are perfectly true' • 'the smell reminded me of French holidays in the sun' • 'my partner could tell the difference if I didn't use it!' • 'this was brilliant: better than all the rest'.

### ✳ ✳ Burt's Bees Carrot Nutritive Body Lotion, £13.50/207ml

**Score: 7.7/10**

Although this cream didn't score quite as highly as some of our other entries, we've included it because we know how many of you care about putting totally natural products on your bodies – rather than creams which are masquerading as natural. This is 98.67 per cent natural, according to Burt's Bees. One tester e-mailed immediately to say that it treated her eczema better than anything her doctor could prescribe; it contains balsam of Peru, an essential oil noted for treating eczema and chapped hands and feet. The antioxidant-rich carrot seed oil undoubtedly works well but some testers weren't keen on the smell or the fact it can stain. Sarah, who is a fan, suggests using it at night or letting it sink in for a few minutes before putting on your nightie or getting in the sheets.

**Comments:** 'Skin immediately felt soft and moisturised, looked dewy and healthy, with a slightly silky shine' • 'the lightest effective body lotion I've ever used: you can put on tights immediately, skintone looks firmer, and it leaves a healthy glow' • 'even used it on my face, and was good under foundation' • 'stopped the itching from eczema where doctor's creams had done nothing' • 'my husband liked the smell, though I didn't' • 'very good pump dispenser'.

**WE ♥ LOVE…**

REN's Wild Yam Omega-7 Body Lotion (see page 152) has a starring role on Jo's bedside table, alongside two 100 per cent natural offerings: Trilogy Nourishing Body Lotion, £14.95/175ml (from a small-but-brilliant New Zealand-based botanical brand that Sarah loves too), and the ultra-rich Softening Body Butter Lemon Zest & Geranium Flower, £22/140g, created by Circaroma, whose products have done very well elsewhere in this book. Jo loves the geranium smell, and the way it makes her feet and elbows feel velvety. Sarah's collection includes Liz Earle's plant-packed Nourishing Botanical Body Cream, £14.50/200ml, Rosa Fina Nourishing Rejuvenating Body Lotion, £21.95/200ml, and the Green People Company's Organic Base Hand & Body Lotion, £10.99/200ml.

# body oils

Oils were the original beauty treats, extracted from nuts, seeds and precious plants since before the time of Cleopatra. They are still ultra-effective today and perfect for last-thing-at-night beautification, when oils can sink in without the risk of spots getting on your clothes

Among these high-scoring choices in this category you'll find lots of all-natural contenders – because oils don't need preservatives. (It's the water in cosmetics that creates a breeding ground for germs.) Interestingly, quite a few testers with skin problems, including eczema and psoriasis, commented how much they improved with regular use of body oils.

### ESPA Detoxifying Body Oil, £24/100ml
**Top Treat**
Score: 8.66/10

ESPA promise this oil can 'combat the effect of toxins, relieve water retention and assist the fight against cellulite' and several of our testers supported this claim vociferously, although they were simply asked to judge its performance as a moisturising body oil. The tangy scent of grapefruit, cypress, juniper berry, lemon and eucalyptus – and the frosted glass jar – were popular.
**Comments:** 'Amazing: already my cellulite has improved vastly, limbs feel firmer, more solid, with

the sponginess gone' • 'loved this! My dry skin feels shiny and moisturised; saggy upper arms better toned in a short time' • 'my decolletage became less dry and crêpey, eczema patches cleared up a treat' • 'definite bloom on my very dry eczema-prone skin' • 'my husband told me I smelt like lemon meringue pie – a compliment, from him!' • 'after a few days my skin was super soft, much more even toned, and quite bright'.

### Elemis Exotic Frangipani Monoi Moisture Melt, £27.50/100ml
Score: 8.16/10

Polynesian women have long used frangipani (monoi) oil to keep their skins supple and sensual. Elemis acknowledge this product may solidify, but can be made liquid – and massage-able – again by placing the bottle in a bowl of warm water. Some testers found this a fiddle, though one loved it, because it was easy to transport.
**Comments:** 'My skin immediately felt smooth and soft and smelt divine' • 'truly my desert island luxury' • 'bright red scaly patches of psoriasis became soft and pinkish in a few days' • 'went on

like silk and made my skin feel incredible; my husband liked the smell, too' • 'a spa treatment in a bottle' • 'very economical' • 'gave wonderful results applied to hands and feet and covered with a warm wrap' • 'also good for cuticles'.

## Nuxe Huile Prodigieuse, £19.50/100ml
### Score 7.68/10

A cult product much-loved by supermodels and make-up artists, Nuxe recommend this spritz-on sinks-in-fast oil for face and hair as well as body. Although it contains no hydrocarbon-derived mineral oils, we didn't feel able to award this a natural 'daisy' as the first four ingredients listed are synthetic ingredients or silicones, which work to smooth skin alongside the product's natural elements of sweet almond, borage, camellia oil, vitamin E and oily extract of hypericum.

**Comments:** 'A "dry" oil that sinks straight into the skin: could dress pretty much immediately; gave body a lovely satiny sheen' • 'skin strokeably soft' • 'great before applying a fake tan' • 'very easy to rub in on small dry areas like elbows, knees and heels' • 'not sticky or oily; left my skin soft and smelt lovely' • 'ideal for all arid body conditions'.

## ❋ ❋ Circaroma Uplifting Skin Serum Bergamot + Purple Sage, £15/28ml
### Score: 7.62/10

This vitamin-rich oil – a blend of sesame, apricot and arnica oils, refreshingly fragranced with essential oils of grapefruit, rosemary, lemon, basil and eucalyptus – provoked unusually mixed responses (with most products, there is a clear consensus): some testers adored it and awarded it ten out of ten; others were less impressed.

**Comments:** '*Loved* this amazing skincare product – like having your own aromatherapist; left me energised (no mean task with a baby) and

uplifted' • 'perfect as a treat for Monday-morning blues' • ' heels softer than they've ever been, scaly legs a bygone, my body looks so sleek – and a heavenly smell' • 'a joy to massage in'.

## *Beauty Steal* Normandie Body Gloss, £4.97/250ml
### Score: 7.5/10

We're delighted our YOU Magazine colleague Normandie Keith's body oil, packaged in a reach-everywhere spritz dispenser, scored so well. Fragranced with mandarin essence, this avocado-oil-based skin spray leaves a silky sheen on skin. (Normandie's very affordable range is available at selected Tesco stores.)

**Comments:** 'My skin looked amazing, very soft and moisturised' • 'my boyfriend said I looked very sexy and smelt divine' • 'my husband adores the lovely light citrus scent' • 'love the feeling of healthy skin – younger, softer and suppler' • 'you don't need much and it took away the really dry skin on the front of my legs and made my arms look really glowy'.

# bust boosters

Most of us could do with a little perkifying in the boob department, we have to admit – and there are creams and lotions designed to do just that. But do they work? Our panels of testers set out to find whether it really is possible to defy gravity

Frankly, we think exercise – and a Wonderbra – can do more for your 'oomph' factor than a cosmetic bust-booster, although they will improve skin condition. Results were mixed: none of these choices impressed all ten panellists who tried them, and not one of the budget buys we trialled scored well enough to be included – so if you really do want to add a bust-booster to your beauty regime, you'll have to splash out. And actually, daily splashes of cold water probably work just as well as pricey products. Frenchwomen swear by it – and so does Sarah.

## tip

According to experts, 80 per cent of us are wearing the wrong size bra, so make an appointment for a fitting in the bra department of a big store or specialist lingerie boutique. You won't regret it.

*Top Treat*

### Sisley Phytobuste, £92/50ml
**Score: 7.5/10**

This lightweight gel – definitely a blow-the-budget buy – is packed with plant and algae extracts, including horsetail, ivy, yarrow and red vine; apply morning and night, in large, circular movements, extending coverage to base of the neck, shoulders and inner arms.

**Comments:** 'The product did appear to work – instantly firming, and my skin feels a lot smoother' • 'seemed to work in lifting and perkiness – a good-textured gel that sinks in fast' • 'skin condition was fantastic – very noticeable; there was a visible sheen if wearing a low-cut top' • 'beautiful fresh fragrance'.

### Elemis Pro-Collagen Lifting Treatment Neck and Bust, £70/50ml
**Score: 6.37/10**

Another luxury choice, this is rich in marine products, including samphire and the brown algae *Padina pavonica*, hand-picked daily by scuba divers off Malta, say Elemis, who clearly believe no effort is too great for our boobs. They add royal jelly, propolis and milk protein to this cream, recommending twice-daily

of ozonic – very pleasant'
• my 'skin looks a lot
younger and healthier
than it did four
weeks ago, mainly
on my neck and
decolleté' • ' skin
tone and firmness
definitely improved,
also on my upper arms'.

### Clarins Bust Beauty Gel, £32.50/50ml
#### Score: 6.18/10

The best-known product in its
category, this offers calming
echinacea, anti-free-radical ginkgo
biloba, ginseng, horsetail, mint and witch hazel.
Clarins recommend applying in the morning for
maximum perking effect.

**Comments:** 'I noticed a marked improvement
– my skin looked firmer, as if I'd had a mini-lift'
• 'definite improvement; felt firmer, skintone
brighter – I've bought it again twice' • 'skin was
smoother and more toned' • 'instant softening;
it made my skin almost luminous'.

application of the product to the entire bust and
neck area for best results.

**Comments:** 'Tone and clarity of skin were
improved, crepiness reduced, and my chest
looks and feels slightly more perky' • 'I felt more
confident wearing lower cut tops – it almost
makes me want to grab the nearest man and
push his head in my cleavage!' • 'smelled kind

# cellulite treatments

A miracle product that melts away lumps and bumps is top of many a beauty wish list. Does it exist? Not exactly, is the verdict of the hundreds of women who've trialled anti-cellulite products for us – but these products do improve the look of 'orange-peel' skin, for at least some of our testers

We ask panellists to try the assigned product over a period of months, on one side of their body, for comparison, and to take before-and-after measurements. As we've often said, we tend to believe that any diligent programme of massage and/or body brushing (see Tip), combined with the use of a good body cream, will deliver comparable benefits – especially when you consider that the winning product – read on – isn't really targeted at cellulite at all.

## WE LOVE…

Even at 40-something-plus – and not exactly Kate Moss thin – we have little need for cellulite products. We think it's because we eat mainly organic food, and drink lots of water, and there's a theory that cellulite is exacerbated by synthetic food additives, pesticides and other chemicals in food: the body doesn't know what to do with them, so it wraps them in fat and stores them in the most convenient spot – the thighs.

## Beauty Steal — Revlon Dry Skin Relief Firming, £3.99/200ml
### Score: 7.42/10

As we've just indicated, the top-scoring product in our cellulite category turns out to be a relatively inexpensive moisturiser, which Revlon put forward for testing in this category because of its firming properties. It features AHA fruit acids, to smooth skin, an antioxidant complex and a bit of sun protection (SPF4 – not enough to rely on). Perhaps unsurprisingly, our testers' consensus was that this was truly impressive for its firming action, less so for its anti-dimpling effect.

**Comments:** 'Smoother, less pitted appearance' • 'skin felt quite smooth and seemed to be a little firmer' • 'skin definitely looked progressively smoother after each application; excellent results – silky skin' • 'my legs did feel smooth' • 'cellulite is less noticeable and less dimpled; skin also feels firmer and looks more even'.

## Clarins Total Body Lift, £28/200ml

**Score: 7.35/10**

This light gel is a new launch from Clarins – clearly Europe's number one in cellulite, with a 33 per cent market share. A 'fat-releasing complex' of geranium, caffeine and cangzhu root extract from China is combined with other somewhat obscure plant extracts – agrimony, *Uncaria tormentosa* and hortonia; Clarins prescribe a new 'Self-Massage Body Contouring Method' of application, to stimulate and drain problem zones.

**Comments:** 'Skin felt soft and tingly straight away, looked much smoother and felt soft; after six weeks, cellulite is definitely better on my thighs – the best anti-cellulite cream I've tried – and I have tried lots' • 'very detailed instructions for application, massage, exercise' • 'texture definitely smoother and more refined'

## ✻ ✻ Elemis Cellutox Active Body Concentrate, £26.50/100ml

**Score: 7.3/10**

For those who prefer a more natural choice, this is a 100 per cent botanical product, essentially a massage oil for problem zones, combining almond, sunflower and vitamin E oils with active botanicals including juniper, sea buckthorn, lemon and sea fennel. NB: it's more appropriate for use at night-time, as it's unctuous and could mark clothes.

**Comments:** 'Very impressed; definitely firmer skin and orange peel has smoothed out' • 'skin felt smoother, less rough' • 'cellulite looked smoother and less dimply' • 'the top of the leg I used this on was slightly less lumpy than the other' • 'a two-minute miracle! Refines, tightens and smooths out any wobbles – treated side looked moderately leaner, with improved skin quality; after six weeks a dramatic difference, with smoother, more toned thighs and cashmere-soft skin, less orange peel; also improved the look of

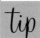 **Buy a body brush!** Test on your forearm before buying to see that the bristles are neither too soft or scratchy. Use it daily on dry skin, as hard as you can on dimply areas, always brushing towards your heart. It really works. Exercise helps too, especially walking and yoga.

my stretch marks' • 'I definitely look and feel firmer, which is good enough for me!'

## ✻ ✻ Decléor Aromessence Contour Slimming Aromatic Fluid, £32.50/200ml

**Score: 6.95/10**

Well, get this: after four years of research, Decléor claim that it's possible to reduce your cellulite simply by breathing in the blend of five essential oils – basil, black pepper, hyssop, grapefruit and clary sage – in this oil. Inhaling this apparently releases noradrenaline, which kick-starts the body to get to work on excess fat reserves. Decléor also suggest a special application technique for this 'non-greasy' oil, which is 100 per cent natural.

**Comments:** 'Lots of easy-to-follow instructions, fabulous moisturiser, at the least; texture of skin very soft and smooth; after six weeks, looks loads smoother and possibly firmer' • 'a lovely fragrant product with results that even my boyfriend noticed: smoother skin, less dimpled, smoother texture, two centimetres reduction in thigh size' • 'very medicinal smell, so you think it must be doing you good' • 'lost an inch, though the cellulite wasn't reduced' • 'thigh looked instantly more toned and cellulite less obvious – as that wore off, skin definitely felt smoother'.

# uplifting bath treats

When our get-up-and-go has got up and gone, sometimes all it takes is a zingy, zesty, energy-boosting bath or shower to help us back on our feet. We asked our panels of testers to trial these when they were feeling exhausted, and on sluggish mornings. One caution, however: the fragrance tends to be potent, for obvious reasons, so wearing scent afterwards may be a bit of a no-no

## WE LOVE...

To our minds, Aromatherapy Associates and Thisworks are in a league of their own when it comes to aromatherapy bath treats: one capful fills not only the bathroom with fragrant air, but the whole house. Jo adores Thisworks Energy Bank (reviewed opposite), alternating it with Aromatherapy Associates Revive Morning Bath & Shower Oil, £27/55ml, which is better than a double espresso at waking her up! And Sarah – a bit boringly – likes exactly the same.

## Top Treat ✿ ✿ Dr Hauschka Rosemary Bath, £14/150ml

Score: 8/10

This totally natural bath oil, from a reasonably priced range based on bio-dynamically grown plants, features warming rosemary. It's so stimulating that Dr Hauschka warn you not to use it at night. Do also try a couple of drops in your morning face washing water, as a wake-up call for the senses.

**Comments:** 'I was very tired but felt invigorated, energised and mood definitely enhanced' • 'skin beautifully soft and supple' • 'I bought three as Christmas presents' • 'my husband said "what a beautiful smell" and uses it himself' • 'very calming, yet I felt warm and energised' • 'almost like a full body beauty treatment'.

## Beauty Steal Champneys Water Mint Stimulating Shower Gel, £5/175ml

Score: 7.87/10

This is actually a moisturising body wash, with a double minty whammy of peppermint and spearmint essential oils plus uplifting orange. While not exactly cheap-cheap, it's the most affordable of those that delivered on their energy-boosting promises.

**Comments:** 'Before shower – tired and sluggish. After shower – uplifted, refreshed and zingy!' • 'my headache which had been nagging me went and I felt much brighter and happier!' • 'my skin felt clean, fresh, smooth and wonderfully silky afterwards' • 'I felt instantly invigorated and knew I was going to have a great night out!' • 'I'm finding this product is slowly addictive'.

## ✻ ✻ Thisworks Energy Bank Bath and Shower Oil, £30/55ml
**Score: 7.55/10**

Our friend Kathy Phillips gave up the beauty directorship of *Vogue* to launch her own range of aromatherapy products, in tandem with Aromatherapy Associates. Our testers raved about this 'energy blockbuster', a fusion of ylang-ylang, patchouli, geranium, sandalwood and rosemary essential oils.

**Comments:** 'Fantastic fragrance, and very natural – I felt uplifted, mentally clear, raring to go!' • 'this is the ultimate pamper product' • 'gorgeous aroma: not too overpowering: instantly invigorating and relaxing all at once' • 'expensive, but it lasts for ages'.

## ✻ ✻ Decléor Aromessence de Bain Aromatic Bath Oil, £41/100ml
**Score: 7.4/10**

This highly concentrated essence has lemon, angelica and lavender essential oils, in a vitamin A-and-E-enriched hazelnut base. Decléor say that the oil does double-duty 'as part of a slimming programme…massaged into specific areas' (but we didn't ask our testers to comment on that).

**Comments:** 'I was stressed and very tired: after bathing I felt more relaxed and revitalised, and my head was cleared of the day's stresses' • 'I would buy this regardless of price' • 'really divine treat: classy bottle, and a fabulous smell' • 'this picked me up when I was drained, tired and lacking sparkle' • 'left my skin smooth to the touch with a slight sheen'.

## Clarins Tonic Bath and Shower Concentrate, £13.50/200ml
**Score: 7.25/10**

This lightly foaming concentrate can be used on a sponge, to lather skin. Its firming, toning, energising action comes from juniper, pine, rosewood, geranium, peppermint and rosemary, so Clarins tell us.

**Comments:** 'Heavenly smell, invigorating and really clean; I was tired and low and it really pepped me up and put me in great party spirits' • 'made my skin smooth and supple' • 'I felt instantly uplifted when I breathed in the vapours' • 'rejuvenating and refreshing'.

## ✻ ✻ Liz Earle Naturally Active Vital Oils Harmony, £8.75/10ml
**Score: 7.1/10**

'Do you crave a sense of balance?' asks the blurb for this oil, which fuses citrus notes like grapefruit, clementine and neroli with grounding frankincense and uplifting rosemary. Frankly, who doesn't?

**Comments:** 'A wonderful energising treat' • 'I went from being totally exhausted to being refreshed, invigorated and energised' • 'my skin felt velvety' 'loved the gentle aroma and my whole house smelt gorgeous' • 'like having a liqueur – smooth and uplifting'.

# relaxing bath treats

At the end of a tough day, we regularly give thanks for the restorative powers of hot water and aromatherapy oils. And so, apparently, do our testers, who lay back and soaked in these blissful bath blends, awarding them some very high marks for their power to de-stress, de-angst (and for smelling di-vine)

Several of the relaxers that our teams trialled are all natural – which, we think, is an issue, if you're going to spend 20 minutes soaking in them. The all-natural products have two 'daisies'.

## ⚜ REN Moroccan Rose Otto Bath Oil, £22.50/150ml
**Score: 9.27/10**

*Top Treat*

Rose Otto is one of the world's priciest and most precious essential oils, and REN (from the Swedish for 'clean') have decanted loads into this oil, accounting for the utterly gorgeous smell.

**Comments:** 'This product is heaven: if there are ten products to try before you die, this is one!' • 'when I feel low, I smell the bottle and that alone lifts me' • 'smelt like my grandmother's rose garden, divine, romantic, old-fashioned' • 'my skin was soft and I felt very relaxed' • 'felt relaxed and rejuvenated' • 'definitely improved my sleep'.

## ⚜⚜ Thisworks Deep Calm Bath & Shower Oil, £30/55ml
**Score: 8.44/10**

We're not surprised that this new oil scored impressively well: you'll find it on our own bathroom shelves (see opposite, 'We Love…'). Made by Aromatherapy Associates for Kathy Phillips's range, it seems pricey until you discover a little really does go a l-o-n-g way – more than 20 baths per bottle, say testers – thanks to the super-high concentration of vetiver, camomile and high-altitude lavender essential oils, in a skin-nurturing pure coconut oil base. (Thisworks Energy Bank Oil also triumphed as an Uplifting Bath Treat – see page 163.)

**Comments:** 'Before: tired, preoccupied – after: tired, relaxed, untroubled!' • 'skin felt wonderfully moisturised' • 'ideal way to unwind after a stressful day, with candles, a good book and *The Archers*' • 'a little certainly went a long way' • 'bath was easy to clean after' • '*fantastic* smell – wafted from the bathroom into the bedroom' • 'I loved the white glass bottle – a fabulous present for a stressed out friend!'

## I Coloniali Relaxing Bath Cream with Bamboo Extract, £11/250ml
**Score: 8.44/10**

Inspired by the Orient and incorporating bamboo extract and moisturising oils, this is a foaming bath cream. Testers loved its soothing silkiness but worried slightly about having a glass jar in a slippery bathroom.

**Comments:** 'A lovely product: smelt fantastic; even my boyfriend stole some' • 'slight foaming – water felt like silk and skin soft after' • 'loved this smell, unusual, like incense' • 'one of the best bath products ever – so relaxing and luxurious'.

### *Beauty Steal* ✿✿ Organic Blue Relaxing Bath and Massage Oil, £7.95/100ml

**Score: 8.42/10**

Hats off to this Soil Association-certified organic product, which is very reasonably priced. With oils of lavender, geranium, Roman camomile and grapefruit in a moisturising base (sunflower, jojoba and coconut) it can double as a massage blend.

**Comments:** 'Loved it; skin felt so soft and didn't need a moisturiser for two days' • 'totally relaxed and calm after using it – wonderful sleep' • 'left me relaxed and clear-headed with soft skin'.

### L'Occitane Lavender Harvest Foaming Bath, £13.50/500ml

**Score: 8.4/10**

The higher the altitude at which the lavender is grown, the finer the fragrance, experts say – and the flowers in this have been harvested from over 800 metres above sea level. Although it contains a chemical (non-drying) detergent, it worked well for one eczema sufferer. This works out less expensively per millilitre than the Organic Blue product – the downside to that, our testers discovered, is that you have to use much more of the product for a similar effect.

**Comments:** 'The smell lingered on my skin, which made me drift off into a soothing sleep' • 'my boyfriend, who suffers from eczema, tried it and found it non-irritating, so I'm going to give it a gold star!' • 'I liked the fact that it is non-drying and non-oily, so I can wash my hair in it as well' • 'my skin felt lovely and really soft after I had used this' • 'this was more than just a bath foam – also quite definitely a mood treatment.'

# body scrubs

Becoming a (body) scrubber is the fast track to skin bliss. Here are the products our testers raved about, in an impressively high-scoring category

For top-to-toe silkiness, exfoliating your body will do far more than mere body lotion ever can: by buffing away the dead cells that sit on the surface (especially around knees, elbows and heels), a good scrub makes skin feel instantly velvety – and it helps your chosen body lotion to sink in much more effectively, too. In fact, some oil-based scrubs do away with the need for body lotion altogether, leaving a veil on the surface after rinsing. One time a body scrub is a beauty must is before self-tanning, ensuring much more even results. But never use a salt-based scrub on just-shaved skin, or if you've been gardening/scratched by the cat; the 'ouch' factor can bring tears to your eyes. Older testers particularly liked this category, commenting that the products made their skin look and feel younger.

## Top Treat
### L'Occitane Delicious Almond Paste, £22.50/200ml
Score: 8.95/10

While we'd never recommend crushed nut shells for exfoliating the face, the pulverised almond grains in this winning scrub combine with sugar crystals, almond oil and almond butter for a rich, thick scrub that does a super-effective job.

**Comments:** 'Skin felt fantastic after, really soothed, firmed and comforted: the most luxurious dreamy product' • 'delicate scrub that left my skin feeling gently polished, not harshly rubbed ' • 'incredible texture: a soft but heavy cream that melts on your skin to become smooth and milky and was easy to rinse off'.

## Clinique Sparkle Skin Body Exfoliating Cream, £16.50/250ml
Score: 8.8/10

The menthol in this rich, creamy blue-green scrub gives a cooling, invigorating sensation, while the rounded jojoba beads and gentle salicylic acid deliver a skin-buffing double whammy. All our testers said they'd buy it.

**Comments:** 'I loved this product, which polishes skin so it's smooth, silky and soft as a baby's bottom' • 'this scrub really cleared my mind as well as making my body tingle and

giving a feeling of increased tone in my legs'
• 'I found that my very dry skin didn't need a
moisturiser if I used this daily' • 'Great packaging,
great smell, great product.'

## Sisley Energizing Foaming Exfoliant for the Body, £25/125ml
**Score: 8.8/10**

This fluid gel lathers with water on the skin into
a fine, creamy foam, with 'polyethylene
microspheres for buffing beads' (that's tiny
particles of plastic, to the rest of us). Essential
oils of rosemary and lavender give an aromatic
fragrance, with horsetail and gentian root extract
to give skin a toned look.

**Comments:** 'Wonderful product: my skin had a
plump dewy look after towelling: it got rid of dry
elbows and plucked chicken skin after one
application; after a week my skin looks as if it's
been airbrushed' • 'I have bad circulation in my
legs and they lack lustre but this really brought a
glow and colour to the skin'.

## Clarins Aroma Body Care Toning Body Polisher, £23.50/250g
**Score: 8.45/10**

Clarins combines Camargue sea salt, white
sugar beet crystals, hazelnut oil and shea butter
with a detoxifying and revitalising blend of mint,
rosemary, rosewood and geranium essential oils
in this moisturising skin-slougher. Our panel
trialled the Toning option; the identical
formulation is also available as a Relaxing Body
Polisher infused with de-stressing essential oils.

**Comments:** 'My skin felt fantastic after using
this – no need for cream. I can't say enough
how much I liked it' • 'amazing, mind-blowing
smell, and over two weeks my skin condition
really improved, feeling smooth and nourished'
• 'real indulgence – it felt as if each grain was

coated in moisturiser' • 'my skin looked perkier
than it has done in years'.

## Bliss Sweet Orange and Spearmint Scrub, £28/345g
**Score: 8.2/10**

This was developed by skin 'guru' Marcia
Kilgore for her heavenly Bliss spas, and is now
available for home use. Testers particularly loved
the sense-zinging mint and orange fragrance.

**Comments:** 'The best body scrub I've ever
used, very moisturising' • 'very easy to use and
wash off: my skin felt alive' • 'this stuff is
fabulous! I felt I had a completely new skin – my
new secret weapon for summer skin survival'
• 'Thanks to using this I now have peachy skin
on my upper arms with no goose pimples and
a babylike soft bum too!'

## Estée Lauder Body Performance Exfoliating Body Polish, £24/200ml
**Score: 8.16/10**

This radiance-boosting formula from Lauder's
state-of-the-art body care range features
moisturising beads with vitamin E .

**Comments:** 'My very dry skin is smoother to
touch, less dry and scaly, and looks healthier
and in better condition' • 'it got rid of all the
pimples on my upper arms in just a few days'
• 'good texture: the small hard granules give

*tip* For a simple DIY scrub,
just mix a teaspoon of salt with
enough organic extra virgin olive
oil (or any other kind of oil, from
sunflower to almond) to make a
runny paste.

a really good scrub, without hurting or irritating the skin' • 'my thighs and bottom look much smoother and more appealing!'

## Darphin Hydrorelax Body Exfoliating Cream, £23/200ml
**Score: 8/10**

This softening product (from a French brand now owned by the Estée Lauder empire) has extracts of bamboo and lotus, fragranced with essential oils of lavender and rose.

**Comments:** 'My rough pimply upper arms felt silky smooth after using this gentle, heavenly smelling exfoliator' • 'smoothed on beautifully – my skin felt wonderful afterwards, and really perked up' • 'really loved using this thick luxurious body cream with tiny blue exfoliating particles' • 'I felt totally pampered'.

### WE LOVE…

Jo's so obsessed with body scrubs there's barely room on the edge of her bath for a rubber duck; favourites include Finders Salt Brushing, £9.99/500g, because you don't need moisturiser afterwards, ESPA Detoxifying Salt Scrub, £25.50/700g, and Champneys Citrus Glow Sugar Scrub, £8.50/350ml. Sarah's eccentric plumbing means scrubs are a no-no, so she is devoted to dry skin body brushing instead.

## Elemis Lime and Ginger Salt Glow, £32.50/410g
**Score: 6.93/10**

This was the most popular of the more natural options with our testers. (It's amazing how many so-called 'natural products' actually turn out to contain ingredients such as propylene glycol or paraffin.) The active ingredients in this formula are sea salt, lime peel and ginger extract in a kukui, camellia and jojoba oil base. Some testers adored this combination, but a couple were less impressed with the texture, which was described as 'sloppy', bringing the average score down. Elemis warn that this product shouldn't be used if you're pregnant.

**Comments:** 'This product looked gorgeous and made me feel *gorgeous*! It has a fabulous texture and smell. My skin felt absolutely amazing after one week's use' • 'my skin is normally very dry but after using this I didn't need to use a moisturiser' • 'skin was smoother and firmer'.

## *Beauty Steal* The Sanctuary Hot Sugar Body Polish, £9.95/400ml
**Score: 6.9/10**

This body polish was the highest scorer with our panellists among the more affordable choices. Massaged into the skin, the self-heating gel in a glass jar has an intriguing warming action to help stimulate the circulation.

**Comments:** 'This product was a dream to use: I found it very easy to apply and wash off – the heat element meant it felt very soothing, and it left my skin moisturised and smooth' • 'there were no dry or dull patches anywhere on my body after using this; my skin felt buffed and ready for applying my next batch of tan' • 'I had no ingrowing hairs after waxing' • 'the bumps that plague my arms are feeling much less raised since I have been using this'.

# natural deodorants

Recently, the safety of chemicals such as parabens and aluminium compounds in deodorants and antiperspirants has been questioned. Many women prefer natural products, including us, even if they're not quite so sweat-blockingly effective as market leaders. Most of our testers were impressed by the following totally natural choices

*Top Treat*

## Dr Hauschka Deodorant Fresh, £8/50ml

**Score: 8/10**

From the famous Dr Hauschka biodynamic natural range, this roll-on in glass packaging is formulated without synthetics, anti-perspirants or anti-bacterial agents. It's available as a herb-scented Fresh version (which our testers tried), and as a Floral version for sensitive skin.

**Comments:** 'By far the best natural product I have found' • 'I ride a motorbike and go to the gym but remained completely dry, with no hint of smell' • 'no white powder or stickiness, and very pleasant inoffensive smell; felt fresh and dry all day and evening' • 'didn't sting after shaving • 'does a very good job of keeping you dry in all conditions' • 'I used this straight after waxing and felt absolutely no pain'.

## Green People Organic Deodorant Gentle Control, £6.49/75ml

**Score: 7.05/10**

This alcohol-free (therefore no-stinging) product, which also avoids pore-clogging aluminium, is based on naturally occurring ammonium alum

to fight germs, which has been combined with zinc ricinoleate (from castor oil) to deodorise, along with olive leaf extract, antiseptic essential oils and floral waters.

**Comments:** 'Ten out of ten for this product which kept me fresh, also dry (surprisingly), through a night out' • 'I stayed totally fresh all day and didn't feel that this was going to have any adverse health effects' • 'I sweated on a long walk but didn't feel sticky or smelly' • 'I was a bit sceptical at first but am now a convert!'

## Jason Aloe Vera Deodorant, £4.99/75g

**Score: 6.8/10**

Packed with skin-soothing and softening aloe vera, this gentle roll-on version also includes vitamin E and camomile extract among the ingredients. However, if you 'glow' a lot, this may not give you the protection you want.

**Comments:** 'A very good product that worked as well as my usual one; kept me fresh and dry through an evening out' • 'no residue or stickiness, and dried quickly enough' • 'this keeps me dry for 12 hours if I don't do brisk exercise' • 'I felt confident with this'.

# hair removers

Shave it, cream it, tweeze it, wax it – there are plenty of ways to tackle unwanted hair on face and body. Our testers are now baby smooth, having worked their way through dozens of depilators to bring you news of the most effective fuzz-busters

Jo's fave fuzz-buster (as mentioned, right) is the Gillette Venus Divine Razor, but in stubbly emergencies she reaches for the Philips Moi Wet & Dry Ladyshave, £30, a rechargeable razor that can even be used in the shower, and looks amazingly stylish – think blue, ergonomic, rubber grip – for an electric razor. Sarah has waxed for decades, literally, and has three hairs under her arms, and so few on her legs that she can either tweeze them off or uses pre-waxed strips, which all work adequately – just do make sure you warm the wax by smoothing them down on the skin with the heel of your hand.

As with every other category, the products were sent to ten women, who reported back in detail, in this case, on pleasure of use – or, often, not – effectiveness, and how long it took hair to re-grow. On the basis of these results, we can honestly say that hair removal technology still has a way to go – meanwhile, this is as close as you can get to no-fuss, no-muss fuzz-busting.

**Top Treat**

## Gillette Venus Divine Razor, £6.65
**Score: 8.67/10**

Because Jo's such a fan of this razor, we decided we'd send it to ten women to see what they thought – and our testers were equally impressed, voting it into first place. With a rubberised grip – for control and comfort when shaving – and intensive moisture strips enriched with aloe and natural oils, the Venus Divine features triple blades, a swivel head and smoothing cushions that gently stretch skin to lift hair for a close, comfortable shave. Refill blades

are available, which makes this a far more planet-friendly option than disposable versions.
**Comments:** 'Excellent! Very impressed. Easy to use, effective and worked just fine with soap and water – though recommended shaving gel – skin very comfortable and smoother than usual, no irritation, cuts or scratches' • 'flexible action enables all nooks and crannies to be accessed: the best woman's razor on the market – somehow makes me feel slimmer' • 'quick to use in the shower, even for a hairy beast' • 'gave a very comfortable close shave – skin wasn't red or cut, the lubricating strips are great' • 'easy to take away'.

 **tip** If you're waxing, try to avoid the run-up to your period, when pain thresholds are lower and the 'ouch' factor much higher. And that applies to salon appointments, too.

### ☀ ☀ Nad's Facial Wand Kit, £13.95
**Score: 7/10**

Nad's was born on the kitchen table of a Sydney mother, inspired by her daughter's unhappiness about dark body hair. Christened a 'no-heat hair removal gel', it's a concoction of fructose, honey, molasses, lemon, vinegar and food dye – for the distinctive green colour – inspired by the ancient Oriental concept of 'sugaring'. This kit – designed to remove eyebrow, chin and lip hair – features ten specifically shaped cotton strips, five sealed 'preparation' towelettes, plus a mirror, so you can see exactly what you're doing.
**Comments:** 'After using this a few times, regrowth was finer' • 'the lip-gloss-style bottle made it very easy to use the gel' • 'I have sensitive skin but this was very easy to use and effective – no soreness or red spots after'.

### ☀ ☀ Nad's Hair Removal Gel, £18.95/6oz
**Score: 6.78/10**

Using the same natural formulation as the facial wand, above, this is for more extensive areas of body hair. As it works at room temperature, there's no chance of burning skin. And – as an

aside – you might like to know that there's now a Nad's kit for men, to tackle hairy backs!
**Comments:** 'Brilliant on legs, bikini line, eyebrows – anywhere!' • 'less painful than traditional waxing, no mess and water-soluble – brilliant!' • 'great for my sensitive skin' • 'the gel really is soluble – unlike wax; painful though' • 'fine stubble returned only after two and a half weeks'.

### Veet Bladeless Razor, £6.99
**Score: 6.29/10**

A slightly weird hybrid of razor and depilatory cream: first, slather on the 'easy-rinse' gel-cream, with hydrating ingredients. Then, when it's dissolved the hair – on legs, underarm or bikini line – scrape off the gunk with a piece of plastic, shaped like a razor. Because the plastic gizmo's bladeless, though, Veet (formerly Immac) point out there's no risk of razor rash, nicks or cuts. Testers found it very efficient but two reported some irritation and several commented on the 'age-old smell of hair-removing creams through the process' – which did of course wear off.
**Comments:** 'Product very easy to spread, removed hair in just three minutes very effectively – skin very soft after removing with the razor tool, which was easy to rinse' • 'made my legs feel incredibly smooth and left a moisturising oil film, which stopped skin drying out' • 'really liked the softness and smoothness of my legs'.

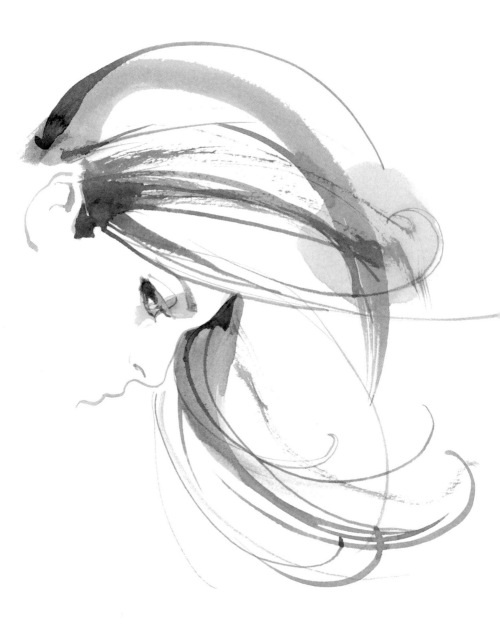

# Hair

8

Shiny, swingy, gleaming – and tameable – hair is on every woman's beauty wish list. But if you're tearing yours out trying to choose the best products from the gazillions out there, we've done the homework for you

# frizz-beaters

Even smooth-haired beauties can turn into Struwwelpeter when the humidity levels rise. And for the 30 per cent of us who cope with dry, frizzy unmanageable hair all the time, frizz-beating products can have a cheering effect on hair confidence – and make a curl do what a curl oughta do

The good news: there really are 'hair management' products out there that tame flyaways, de-frizz and also define curls, if you so choose. For this book, our testers spritzed and smoothed their way through plenty of new launches, but only one, Paul Mitchell, joined the ranks of our previous winners, which are still real hair heroes – and real steals, in some cases.

### Top Treat — Aveda Light Elements Smoothing Fluid, £19.50/100ml
### Score: 8.8/10

At the heart of the Light Elements™ range is certified organic lavender water, traditionally used in aromatherapy for its anti-bacterial properties, found here alongside organic jojoba oil, to help moisturise and condition, in a lightweight fluid. Several of our ten testers – not all with dry and/or frizzy hair – gave it full marks.

**Comments:** 'The best product I've ever used on my long, highlighted, fluffy hair – totally lives up to its promises: hair is soft, manageable, bouncy, smoother and glossier' • 'incredibly easy to use; gorgeous smell' • 'de-frizzers tend to make my wavy slightly frizzy hair lank – this left it soft, manageable and very shiny' • 'excellent for use with irons' • 'left no residue' • 'good for defining layers in straight layered hair' • 'easy to spread on wet or dry hair; brilliant on all my family's different sorts of hair – the best styling agent ever'.

## WE LOVE...

Jo is delighted to report that frizzy hair is one of the few beauty woes she doesn't have! Nor does Sarah, except in really humid conditions, when she uses a spot of Aveda Light Elements Smoothing Fluid (right).

## Kérastase Oléo-Relax Discipline Serum, £14.10/125ml

**Score: 8.78/10**

The Oléo-Relax range – available exclusively through Kérastase salons – has been created to deliver 'long-lasting anti-frizz control, natural softness, smoothness and amazing shine'. This pump product contains a 'unique Nutri-Huile complex' from shorea oil and palm tree oil, together with UV filters for protection.

**Comments:** 'Very good de-frizz factor; hair softer and smoother than ever before' • 'fantastic for my fine, flyaway hair' • 'my hair used to frizz a lot in wet weather; now so well behaved!' • 'immediate shine – great for a busy schedule' • 'my new miracle hair product for my thick curly hair'.

## Paul Mitchell Super Skinny Serum, £11.50/150ml

**Score: 8.62/10**

Paul Mitchell say this contains a 'unique smoothing complex which penetrates into the hair shaft, where it helps to displace water', and thermal protectors to guard against damage from heated styling tools.

**Comments:** 'Very easy to apply; no stickiness – went through damp hair easily' • 'less frizz after blow-drying; hair more shiny, but not oily; didn't weigh it down – great to use' • 'let my frizz-prone hair dry naturally after washing into soft curls, rather than the usual fingers-in-the-socket effect' • 'hair kept its shape a lot better' • 'I have an oily scalp but this left hair light with a lot of movement'.

##  Garnier Fructis Sleek & Shine Weightless Smoothing Serum, £3.99/150ml

**Score: 8.3/10**

Sleek & Shine comes from a range that is targeted at coarse, dry rebellious hair. Based on vitamin-enriched micro oils from apricot kernels

L'Oréal 'face' Dayle Haddon carries in her handbag a silk scarf at all times – Hermès, actually, reports Jo – whips it out and ties it on her wavy hair when there's the merest hint of drizzle in the air. Keeping off moisture is the secret of smooth hair, she insists.

and avocado, this high-scoring budget product is an ultra-light, leave-in formula.

**Comments:** 'Fantastic – my long, naturally wavy, slightly frizzy hair felt smooth, silky and looked sleek – excellent for styling with dryer' • 'I'm a big fan – better value than similar ones, and turns frizz into curls' • 'this was superb for my very coarse, curly, frizzy, greying, coloured hair; I will definitely be changing to this'.

##  Elvive Smooth-Intense Serum, £5.99/100ml

**Score: 7.77/10**

Elvive's Smooth-Intense products contain a silicone derivative and camilina oil to nourish, detangle and smooth. Three L'Oréal winners in this category – Garnier Fructis and Kérastase are also both L'Oréal divisions – clearly make them the Kings of Smooth Hair.

**Comments:** 'This was excellent – my slightly wavy long hair was shinier and sleeker, with very little frizz' • 'my highlighted, quite dry, frizzy hair stayed smooth after using this, even in damp conditions' • 'found it much easier to straighten my hair with irons – and the effect was even better, when I used it with matching conditioner'.

# hair masks

Every hairdresser we've ever interviewed has prescribed a once-a-week deep treatment to combat the damage caused by hairdriers and heated styling tools, colouring products and UV light. So our panels of testers treated their stressed tresses with a selection of deep conditioners and hair masks – and liked these best

In a perfect world, you'd apply a hair mask for 20 to 30 minutes, once or twice a week. But in an imperfect world, hair masks should at least be part of your summer beauty regime: these intensive conditioners are the best way to prep hair before it's subjected to the beach, the pool, or a jaunt in a convertible car/speedboat. We've given this category lots of space because so many products scored so well, and – indulgently – because we just love and believe in hair masks! NB: as Jo's colourist Susan Baldwin – at John Frieda – points out, 'When it comes to hair masks, more is more.' So be generous.

**tip**

We don't eat microwaved food – but we do like the way a microwave warms up a hair mask, encouraging it to penetrate further into thirsty hair. Hair should be towel-dried before applying a mask; once that's done, head for the kitchen: dollop your mask into a bowl, set the timer for ten seconds – remove and slather on. Leave as long as possible, then rinse. Hey, presto – super-shiny hair!

*Top Treat*

## Lancôme Hair Nutrition Intense Extra Rich Conditioning Mask, £18/200ml

**Score: 8.25/10**

Incredibly rich and luscious, this winning creamy honey-coloured mask repairs dried and damaged fibres with a blend of hair-repairing agents that Lancôme call 'Nutri-Complexe™'. Interestingly, it worked well on all different types of hair, according to our testers' reports.

**Comments:** 'This product worked so well on my thick wavy slightly frizzy hair: very simple to use – just five minutes on towel-dried hair, lovely smell, rich texture, and easy to work through; made my hair smoother, silkier, shinier – easier to blow-dry; excellent for calming frizz' • 'hair was shiny glossy even after blowdrying; my coloured hair tends to be tuggy after washing, so I use a leave-in conditioner, but this made it very soft and easy to dry: didn't need my usual serum or smoothing balm' • 'a real treat for coloured, over-processed hair like mine' • 'didn't weigh down my fine hair, or make it greasy: excellent' • 'smoothed split ends; hair appeared more nourished and healthy looking'.

## TIGI Self-Absorbed Mega-Vitamin Conditioner, £8.70/250ml
Score: 8.2/10

According to TIGI, this 'pumps hair full of body and shine!' They claim it also tames static, smooths dry ends and is great for working out messy tangles, but although most of our testers loved this mega-vitamin formula, it didn't suit absolutely everyone.

**Comments:** 'Delicious smelling – my husband said how gorgeous my hair smelt; hair looked extremely shiny and was a lot easier to comb through and style' • 'very simple to apply; no tangles, easy to brush, less frizz' • 'after I left this on for five minutes, my hair had a "just stepped out of the salon" feel' • 'left me with fantastically shiny hair, really easy to comb through' • 'hair looks healthy, shiny and sleek, and I feel well groomed' • 'this was excellent for my long, fine-ish hair; I get through loads of conditioner and this one really stood out'.

## Redken All Soft Heavy Cream, £14.50/250ml
Score: 8.05/10

Another high-scoring product, this time 'ideal for very dry, thick, wiry, coarse hair in need of moisture and control', as Redken explain, though our straight-haired testers also found it to be

## WE ♥ LOVE…

Jo has tried literally every hair mask under the sun, and ever since Estée Lauder, in their wisdom, withdrew their sensational Herbal Hair Pack, alternates between Aveda Damage Control and Frederic Fekkai Protein RX Conditioning Mask, both winners here. When she can get to Paris, she stocks up on Christophe Robin's amazingly re-glossing, wheatgerm-based Intensive Nourishing Treatment for Coloured Hair – you can find it at the boutique Colette – which works wonders on her bleached-to-high-heaven hair. And if she gets the chance – which is not very often! – she likes to book in for a Kérastase ritual, at a Kérastase salon. Sarah's another mask devotee for her very thick, long, coloured hair, loving both Aveda Damage Control and the Christopher Robin product, like Jo; also Phytokarité Ultra Nourishing Conditioner with Shea Butter, £16.50/200ml – cousin to Phytocitrus, overleaf – and Kérastase Reflect Rich Radiance Enhancing Masque, £22/200ml.

fabulous, and fairly weightless. Among the gloss-boosting ingredients to be found in this five-to-15-minute hair pack are avocado oil, glycerine and wheat proteins.

**Comments:** 'This was the best product of all the ones I tried – just fantastic; after use my straight hair was silky and light' • 'my hair looked healthier and brighter' • 'my hairdresser says this is one of the best conditioners he's used; has a superb de-frizz factor' • 'gave instant gloss that earned me compliments' • 'nice, clean scent'.

## ☀ Aveda Damage Remedy Intensive Restructuring Treatment, £18/125ml
### Score: 8/10

Aveda tell us 'this intensely moisturising formula is powered by certified organic ingredients', including quinoa protein, sandalwood, barley extracts, antioxidant sea buckthorn and alfalfa leaf powder, with a relaxing fragrance blended from essential oils of bergamot, mandarin and ylang-ylang. What's more, you have the option of enjoying this product as part of an Aveda in-salon treatment, complete with scalp massage – or you can plump for the DIY version, if you prefer, which was the one our testers tried.

**Comments:** 'This was lovely! Changed my dry frizzy hair to sleek and shiny' • 'excellent to work through my long hair: gave a lovely gloss and more body to hair, and it stayed in place – at long last! Also, I was able to go an extra day without washing it; didn't weigh it down at all' • 'combing it through my very fine hair was just a dream and gloss was fantastic' • 'lovely scent, smelt refreshing and of essential oils' • 'this was truly a miracle: made my very fine straight hair feel slinky as if it had been professionally blow-dried; it usually looks awful the day after shampooing but this really made a difference'.

## Frederic Fekkai Protein Rx Reparative Treatment Mask, £23/5.5oz
### Score: 8/10

Drop-dead-gorgeous Provence-born Frederic Fekkai is the must-visit hairdresser for Manhattan's ladies who lunch – but he's not just a pretty face, having created some truly impressive luxury haircare. Designed for weak or broken hair, this jar of deep conditioner is enriched with a complex of soy and milk proteins, with a sense-soothing caramel vanilla scent.

**Comments:** 'Fantastic deep conditioning treatment; a small amount really does leave my coarse – much abused – hair beautifully smooth and sleek; almost as good as when my hairdresser does it' • 'lovely vanilla smell, almost good enough to eat' • 'wicked: fabulous gloss, knocks spots off my usual mega-intensive conditioner; loved using it – and the small-ish pot lasted for quite a long time' • 'my 25-year-old daughter with natural brown hair absolutely raved about the gloss and bounce' • 'fabulous: left my hair incredibly soft and shiny, more bouncy and springy, and brightened colour'.

## ☀ Phytologie Phytocitrus Hair Mask, £16.50/200ml
### Score: 8/10

From the French botanical hair specialists Phyto comes this deep tress-treat crammed with natural ingredients, including sweet almond protein, grapefruit extract and shea butter, designed to 'revitalise hair left dry by colouring and perming', by eliminating any alkaline residues which remain. They claim it works its magic in just two to five minutes.

**Comments:** 'Made my recently coloured hair feel thicker and glossy; it also looked brighter' • 'only needed a dime-sized dollop' • 'my thick long hair was smooth and controllable'.

## L'Oréal Paris Elvive Nutri-Ceramide Deep Repair Masque, £3.99/200ml

**Score: 8/10**

This deeply nourishing mask contains a concentrate of micro-nutrients that L'Oréal claim will repair even very dry, damaged hair, restoring it to gloss, smoothness and manageability. Our testers were certainly impressed.

**Comments:** 'Within one hour of using this product, my hair looked as if it had been expertly styled – it hadn't – and stayed that way for over three days' • 'aromatic smell of lemon, grapefruit and pineapple' • 'hair felt incredibly soft and manageable after drying; movement was lovely' • 'reduced the static in my hair' • 'I've been using this for two weeks now, and the condition of my hair is great – what a shine!'.

## MOP C System Reconstructing Treatment, £10.95/200ml

**Score: 8/10**

In a very stylish orange bottle, find this zestily orange-fragranced creation from a loved-by-the-stars brand, containing a mega-dose of vitamin C from papaya, grapefruit, mandarin, mango, lime and lemon – although overall, it's not quite as natural as those ingredients might suggest. One tester gave it 110 marks out of ten!

**Comments:** 'By the end of winter, my hair usually feels lacklustre, dry and brittle; after this treatment it feels like *hair* again – in fact, I'd say it was as good as having a professional treatment' • 'an excellent product that leaves hair glossy and manageable' • 'this is a life-changingly good conditioner – truly amazing; I was having a nightmare coping with new-grey-hair-trauma, and this fixed it – will buy *all* their products, and shares in the company' • 'particularly love the cheeky orange packaging'.

# hair mousses

No hair product delivers va-va-volume, body and hold to hair like styling mousse. But some mousses let hair move, swing and leave it glossy and gleaming, while others make it look dull – or, worse, result in 'helmet head' or 'snowflake scalp'. Read this, and you'll know which to head for

> **tip** The key with successful mousse application, so say our professional hairdresser pals, is to distribute it from root to tip. Squirt an egg-sized mound of mousse into your palm, rub palms and fingers together, then work right through hair. Continue styling, with a drier and brush, or fingers. Some stylists suggest you towel- or blow-dry hair till it's around 70 per cent dry before applying the mousse.

### *Beauty Steal* Trevor Sorbie Rejuvenate Volumising Mousse, £3.99/250ml

**Score: 7.66/10**

Why call it Rejuvenate? Because Trevor Sorbie created this range specifically to tackle the problems of ageing hair, which tends to be thinner and finer, so volume is lost. This light, non-sticky mousse offers cashmere and silk proteins to restore thickness and shine, with panthenol for elasticity, and an antioxidant complex to guard against environmental damage.

**Comments:** 'Has converted me back to mousse as a styling product: impressive!' • 'easy to dispense right amount; easy to comb through hair, or use fingers; reduced frizz and increased shine; hair looked healthier' • 'hair still felt bouncy and fresh at the end of the day' • 'style held really well, without any stickiness or stiffness' • 'hair felt silky soft and very groomed; style lasted all day' • 'held hair in place all day without stiffness or lankness' • 'lovely smelling, non-sticky, easier to blow-dry, gave a lot of body and shine' • 'think this would work on fine hair at all ages'.

### ✻ Aveda Phomollient, £11/200ml

**Score: 7.33/10**

Congratulations to Aveda, who have scored consistently well in every hair category in this book. A non-aerosol product, this froths up when you press the pump, using 'air-infused technology' to build body, detangle and add weightless volume, with a light-to-medium hold. Certified organic ingredients in the formula include shine-enhancing honey, burdock to condition the scalp and smoothing marshmallow root.

**Comments:** 'Made my hair calmer, thicker and fuller; like the way it wasn't sticky and that there are no artificial chemicals' • 'gave a volume that held all day' • 'no tangles, easier to style; liked the honey scent, not too sweet' • 'simple to work through hair with fingers or a comb, easy to blow-dry and style, style held all evening; lasts months, even using daily' • 'really good: can use on wet hair to add volume and shine; leaves hair completely natural, with no stickiness or stiffness; also great for sorting out dry slept-on hair quickly in the morning; doesn't seem to build up on hair at all, and it's not full of chemicals' • 'lovely to feel my tired thin hair feel stretchy and bendy again' • 'I rarely buy styling products but would buy this'.

### *Beauty Steal* L'Oréal Paris Elvive Styliste Curl Control Mousse, £3.49/200ml

**Score: 7/10**

A rich and creamy mousse for long-lasting hold, targeted at the 54 per cent of women with wavy or curly hair, L'Oréal infuse this with Hydra-Proteins, which they describe as an innovative and intensely nourishing compound that protects and boosts curls, adding body, bounce and suppleness to curls without affecting the hair's shine.

**Comments:** 'Perfect for my curly hair, seemed to make it dry quicker and in shape, curls were well defined, light and full of volume' • 'hair is a bit fine and flyaway but this made it seem more "together", smooth, and manageable ' • 'easy to get correct amount; nice fresh scent, easy to work through hair and style; no grease or stickiness – style lasted all evening' • 'really gave volume, but hair

felt very light, didn't have to wash it daily, although style dropped considerably – probably best on shorter hair' • 'firm, light and easy to distribute through hair; really like the fresh clean smell'.

### *Beauty Steal* L'Oréal Paris Elvive Styliste Non-Stop Volume, £3.49/200ml

**Score: 6.75/10**

L'Oréal recommend applying this non-sticky mousse to wet hair, insisting it will guarantee a style 'that has maximum volume but natural hold, making it light and beautiful' – to which we add the following testers' comments…

**Comments:** 'Very easy to apply, pleasantly scented, hair more manageable and easier to style, great additional volume, long-lasting – held style all day' • 'manufacturer promised strength, volume and long-lasting hold, and I would definitely agree' • 'my dry hair felt full and sexy after this; lasted all day and all evening' • 'did an excellent job on blowdrying, and didn't need to use straighteners to smooth out my bob – didn't go flyaway – lived up to promise; gives body and rootlift' • 'takes a bit longer to dry hair upside down, and then with a round radial brush as instructed, but worth it for the full bouncy finish'.

# hair waxes

A far cry from grandpa's hair pomade, waxes enable us to create the textured, mussed-up, choppy styles that have been in hair fashion for the last few years

**WE LOVE…**

Since Jo's likely to have a version of her funky-chunky John Frieda hairdo for the rest of her days, hair waxes are her finishing-touch must-have – and on her bathroom shelf you'll find **John Frieda Sheer Blonde Spun Gold Shaping & Highlighting Balm, £3.95/35g,** and **John Masters Bourbon Vanilla & Tangerine Hair Texturizer, £21/57g,** an all-organic pomade which smells almost good enough to eat. Sarah's long hair doesn't lend itself to waxes.

Although we tested vats of these styling products – well, the equivalent of – few inspired our *Handbag Beauty Bible* panellists to, er, wax lyrical, although each product here had some firm fans. Still, it seems as if the haircare industry has yet to invent the perfect hair wax – but for now, check these out. As for the 'how to'? You only need a tiny touch of product, as a little invariably goes a long way: put a dab on your palm, rub your hands together to coat then, then run through hair, twirling the ends for extra definition. You can always add more if that's not enough, but it's impossible to take these products away without washing hair, if you're too heavy-handed.

*Top Treat*

## Aveda Light Elements Defining Whip, £15/4.2fl oz
**Score: 7.55/10**

Inspired by Japanese technology, this lightweight, whipped wax separates and defines hair, offering a medium hold. It features certified organic lavender water, marshmallow root and organic flaxseed and has a 100 per cent certified organic aroma blend of grapefruit, peppermint, lavender and ylang-ylang. Personally, we're also impressed by the sky-blue packaging, which has a 50 per cent post-consumer recycled content. **Comments:** 'Felt my hair looked its best after using this product' • 'like putting whipped cream through your hair, lovely and light, not sticky, gave my hair shine, which is a miracle' • 'lovely scent, distinctly Aveda; broke hair up softly; works very well in defining and controlling without making hair "claggy"' • 'less fluffy: smooth and shiny' • 'only need a small amount; great on my straight layered hair; created lasting volume – great for defining with no stickiness or flaking' • 'great for fine hair' • 'gave more body, no frizzies, no stickiness or greasiness' • 'created definition and texture without weighing down, just as Aveda claim'.

### ✳ ✳ Phytopro Ultra Gloss Wax,
£9.50/75g
**Score: 7.25/10**

Phyto, the French botanical haircare company, recently created a new range of styling products, in which you'll find this wax serum, designed to give texture and 'character' to hair. Each product in the styling range features myrrh – a natural resin – alongside moisturising pro-vitamin B5, ginseng, vitamin E and a UV filter.

**Comments:** 'Love this: made my hair incredibly shiny and "vital", the healthiest it's ever looked' • 'left hair smooth and sleek' • 'Shine was good; would buy again as a finishing product' • 'very easy to work through hair, made my hair easier to style, left it beautifully shaped, tousled but very tidy, didn't weigh it down – lasted all day' • 'best product for my fine, straight hair by far; gave body and style, movement, texture and manageability'.

### Paul Mitchell Slick Works, £7.50/100ml
**Score: 7.15/10**

Paul Mitchell call this a 'finishing polish' and recommend it for fine-to-medium or chemically treated hair, to help create form and definition while boosting shine. Unlike most of the wax-style products that we trialled for these pages, this is water based, so it shampoos out

**Hair waxes work as an alternative to brow gel, if you have unruly brows: just apply the teensiest touch to your fingertips, rub them together and skim one finger across each brow.**

easily – and it's available exclusively through Paul Mitchell approved salons.

**Comments:** 'Ideal for my very fine short hair, lightweight, easy to use; hair was brilliantly kept in place' • 'I like a more funky look: this did it for me' • 'distributed easily through dry hair' • 'hair was much more manageable; style lasted all day and evening' • 'I have very curly hair but this reduced frizz and made curls more defined and bouncy, left hair feeling soft, style held all day' • 'feels like it's going to be really sticky but wasn't'.

### *Beauty Steal* Charles Worthington Stay Smooth Lasting Impressions Defining Wax, £4.29/50ml
**Score: 6.95/10**

At the affordable end of the spectrum, this is a 'non-greasy' creation by our hairdresser friend Charles Worthington, to 'add shape, separation or definition to newly-smoothed tresses'.

**Comments:** 'Really easy to rub in your hands then smooth over hair; gave a definite hold when I brushed my hair into place, gave a more defined, glossy texture' • 'takeaway size tin is great for travelling; economical – a pea-sized blob is plenty' • 'went on perfectly when warmed between my palms; very easy to work through hair; smoothed and defined hair, looked thicker' • 'hair easier to style and more inclined to shape well, without greasiness or stickiness; completely natural look'.

# DIRECTORY

**Aesop**, available at Liberty's
tel: 020 7734 1234, ext 2225,
www.aesop.net.au

**Alberto VO5**, available nationwide

**Almay**, tel: 0800 085 2716, www.boots.com

**Ambre Solaire**, available at Boots
nationwide, www.boots.com

**Aromatherapy Associates**, tel: 020 8569 7030,
www.aromatherapyassociates.com

**Aveda**, tel: 0870 034 2380, www.aveda.com

**Balm Balm**, www.balmbalm.com

**Barbara Daly**'s make-up for Tesco, available
nationwide, tel: 0800 505 555

**BareEscentuals**, tel: 0870 850 6655,
www.skin-health.co.uk

**Barefoot Botanicals**, tel: 01273 823 031,
www.barefoot-botanicals.com

**Bastien Gonzalez**, for appointments
tel: 020 7565 0869, www.bastiengonzalez.com,
products available at SpaceNK,
tel: 020 8740 2085, www.spacenk.com

**Becca**, tel: 020 7629 9161,
www.beccacosmetics.com

**Benefit**, tel: 0901 113 0001,
www.benefitcosmetics.com

**BioCare**, tel: 0121 433 3727,
www.biocare.co.uk

**Biotherm**, tel: 0800 037 1020

**BKamins** chemist full skincare range is
available in UK at John Bell & Croyden,
London W1, tel: 020 7935 5555

**Bliss**, tel: 0808 100 4151,
www.blisslondon.co.uk

**Bobbi Brown**, tel: 0870 034 2566,
www.bobbibrowncosmetics.com

**Body Shop**, tel: 01903 844 554,
www.thebodyshopinternational.com

**Boots**, tel: 0845 070 8090,
www.boots.com

**Botanics**, tel: 0845 070 8090,
www.boots.com

**Bourjois**, tel: 0800 269 836,
www.bourjois.co.uk

**Burt's Bees**, available at John Lewis or
Harvey Nichols nationwide,
tel: 0845 604 9049/020 7235 5000

**Carita**, tel: 020 7313 8780,
www.carita.co.uk

**Caudalie**, tel: 020 7304 7038,
www.caudalie.com

**Champney's**, tel: 0800 636 262,
www.champneys.co.uk

**Chanel**, tel: 020 7493 3836,
www.chanel.co.uk

**Charles Worthington**, tel: 0845 070 8090, www.charlesworthington.com

**China Glaze**, tel: 020 8979 7261, www.jica.com

**Christian Dior**, tel: 01932 233 909, www.dior.com

**Christophe Robin**, www.colorist.net

**Circaroma**, tel: 020 7359 1135, www.circaroma.com

**Clarins**, tel: 0800 036 3558, www.clarins.co.uk

**Clinique**, tel: 0870 034 2566, www.clinique.co.uk

**Corn Silk**, for mail order and stockists tel: 0239 262 0100

**Crabtree & Evelyn**, tel: 020 7361 0499, www.crabtree-evelyn.co.uk

**Creative Nails**, tel: 0113 216 2994, www.creativenaildesign.com

**Crème de la Mer**, tel: 0870 034 2566

**Cutex**, available nationwide

 **Danièle Ryman**, available at Boots nationwide, www.boots.com

**Darphin**, tel: 01730 232 566

**Decléor**, tel: 020 7313 8780, www.decleor.co.uk

**Dermalogica**, tel: 0800 591 818, www.dermalogica.co.uk

**Dove**, available nationwide, www.dove.com

**Dr Baumann**, tel: 0845 833 5505

**Dr Hauschka**, tel: 01386 792 642, www.drhauschka.co.uk

**DuWop**, available at www.hqhair.com

 **Elemis**, tel: 01278 727 830, www.elemis.com

**Elizabeth Arden**, tel: 020 7574 2722, www.elizabetharden.com

**ESPA**, tel: 01252 352 230, www.espaonline.com

**Essie**, tel: 020 8906 9090, www.perfectnails.uk.com

**Estée Lauder**, tel: 0870 034 2566, www.esteelauder.co.uk

**Eve Lom**, tel: 020 8740 2085, www.spacenk.com

**Evian**, tel: 020 8979 7261, www.jica.com (available at Boots, leading chemists and department stores)

**Frederic Fekkai**, tel: 020 8740 2085, www.spacenk.com

# G

**Garnier**, available nationwide, www.garnierfructis.com

**Gillette**, available nationwide, www.gillettevenus.com

**girl2go**, tel: 01242 225 720, www.girl2go.co.uk (available nationwide at Boots, Sainsbury's and Debenhams)

**Givenchy**, tel: 01932 233 909, www.givenchy.com

**Green People**, tel: 01444 401 444, www.greenpeople.co.uk

**Guerlain**, tel: 01932 233 909, www.guerlain.com

**Guinot**, tel: 01344 873 123, www.rrobson.co.uk

# H

**Healthspan Nurture**, tel: 0800 072 9510, www.healthspan.co.uk/nurture

# I

**I Coloniali**, www.jandeatkinsons.co.uk

**i.d. BareEscentuals**, tel: 0870 850 6655, www.skin-health.co.uk

**Imedeen**, tel: 0845 602 1704, www.imedeen.co.uk

# J

**Jane Iredale**, tel: 020 8450 7111, www.janeiredale.com

**Jason**, available at health and natural food stores nationwide, tel: 0845 072 5825

**Jelly Pong Pong**, www.jellypongpong.com

**Jenny Jordan** eyebrow and make-up clinic, 22 Englands Lane, Belsize Park, London NW3 4TG, tel: 020 7483 2222, www.jennyjordan.com or email jenny@jennyjordan.com

**Jessica**, tel: 020 8381 7793

**Jica**, tel: 020 8979 7261, www.jica.com

**Jo Malone**, tel: 020 7720 0202, www.jomalone.co.uk    *p. 153*

**John Frieda**, tel: 020 7851 9800, www.johnfrieda.com

**John Masters**, tel: 020 7318 3538, www.johnmasters.co.uk

**Johnson's** by Johnson & Johnson, tel: 0845 601 2261, www.jnj.com

**Jurlique**, tel: 0870 770 0980, www.jurlique.co.uk

# K

**Kérastase**, tel: 0800 316 4400

**Kerry Warn**, International Creative Consultant for the John Frieda Professional Haircare division of Kao Brands Company, tel: 020 7851 9800, www.johnfrieda.com

**Kiehl's**, tel: 020 7240 2411, www.kiehls.com

**Korres**, tel: 020 7581 6455, www.korres-natural-products.co.uk

L La Prairie, mail order from Selfridges, tel: 0870 837 7377

Lancaster, tel: 0800 376 0688

Lancôme, available at Boots and major department stores nationwide, www.lancome.co.uk

Laura Mercier, mail order from Selfridges, tel: 0870 837 7377

Lavera, tel: 01557 870 203, www.lavera.co.uk

Leighton Denny Nails at the Urban Retreat at Harrods, tel: 020 7893 8333 and Urban Hair and Beauty at Harvey Nichols Manchester, tel: 0161 828 8856, www.urbanretreat.co.uk

Liz Earle Naturally Active Skincare, mail order, tel: 01983 813 913, www.lizearle.com

L'Occitane, tel: 020 7907 0301, www.loccitane.com

L'Oréal, nationwide, www.lorealparis.co.uk

Lush, tel: 01202 668 545, www.lush.com

M MAC, tel: 020 7534 9222, www.maccosmetics.com

Malibu, tel: 020 8758 0055, www.malibusun.com

Marks & Spencer, 0845 302 1234, www.marksandspencer.com

Max Factor, available nationwide, www.maxfactor.com

Miss Sporty, available at Boots and Superdrug nationwide

Mister Mascara, tel: 020 7237 1007

Model Co, available at SpaceNK nationwide, www.modelco.com.au

Molton Brown, tel: 0808 178 1188, www.moltonbrown.co.uk

MOP, tel: 01282 613 413, www.mopproducts.com

 Nad's, tel: 0870 728 0683, www.nads.com

Nails Inc tel: 020 7382 9353, www.nailsinc.com

Nair, available nationwide at Boots, major supermarkets and independent chemists, www.naircare.co.uk

Nars, mail order from Selfridges, tel: 0870 837 7377

Neal's Yard Remedies, tel: 0845 262 3145, www.nealsyardremedies.com

Nivea, available nationwide, www.nivea.co.uk

Normandie, tel: 0800 505 555, available at Tesco stores nationwide

Nuxe, tel: 01932 827 060, available at selected department stores and leading Boots stores

**O** **OPI**, tel: 01923 240 010,
www.lenawhite.co.uk

**Olay**, available nationwide,
www.olay.com

**Organic Blue**, tel: 020 8424 8844,
www.organicblue.com

**Origins**, tel: 0800 731 4039,
www.origins.com

**P** **Paul & Joe**, available at
Harrods, tel: 020 7730 1234 or
Fenwick, tel: 020 7629 9161,
www.paul-joe-beaute.com

**Paul Mitchell**, tel: 01296 390 590,
www.paulmitchell.com

**Pennyhill The Spa**, tel: 01276 486 100,
www.thespa.uk.com

**Perfect 10**, tel: 020 8573 9907

**Philips (electrical)**, tel: 020 7355 3666,
www.philips.com

**Philosophy**, tel: 0870 990 8452,
www.philosophy.com

**Phyto**, tel: 020 7620 1771,
www.phyto.com

**Phytomer**, tel: 0808 100 2204,
www.thebeautyroom.com

**Pixi**, tel: 020 7287 7211,
www.pixibeauty.com

**Pout**, tel: 020 7379 0379,
www.pout.co.uk

**Prescriptives**, tel: 0870 034 2566,
www.prescriptives.com

 **Redken**,
tel: 0800 444 880

**REN**, tel: 0845 225 5600,
www.renskincare.com

**Revlon**, tel: 0800 085 2716,
www.revlon.com

**Rimmel**, www.rimmellondon.com

**Rosa Fina**, tel: 0870 220 2273,
www.barefoot-botanicals.com

**Ruby & Millie**, available at Boots
nationwide, www.boots.com

**S** **Sainsbury's** Active Natural,
tel: 0800 636 262,
www.sainsburys.co.uk

**St Ives**, available nationwide

**St Tropez**, tel: 0115 983 6363,
www.beautysourceltd.com

**Sally Hansen**, tel: 01276 674 000,
www.sallyhansen.co.uk

**Seche**, tel: 020 8906 9090,
www.perfectnails.uk.com

**Sexy Hair**, tel: 020 8381 7793

**Shavata**, tel: 020 8997 1089

**Shiseido**, tel: 020 7313 4774,
www.shiseido.co.uk

**Shu Uemura**, tel: 020 7235 2375

**Simple**, tel: 0121 327 4750,
www.keep-life-simple.com

**Sisley**, tel: 020 7491 2722,
www.sisley-cosmetics.com

**Skin Benefits**, tel: 020 8559 8244,
www.amirose.com

**Smashbox**, tel: 0800 504 030,
www.qvcuk.com

**Soltan**, tel: 0845 070 8090,
www.boots.com

**Space NK**, tel: 020 8740 2085,
www.spacenk.com

**Stila**, tel: 0870 034 2566

T **T LeClerc**, tel: 020 7629 9161,
www.t-leclerc.com

**The Sanctuary**, available at Boots
nationwide, www.thesanctuary.co.uk

**ThisWorks**, tel: 0845 230 0499,
www.thisworks.com

**Tigi**, tel: 0870 330 0955,
www.tigihaircare.co.uk

**Trevor Sorbie**, tel: 01372 375 435,
www.trevorsorbie.com

**Trilogy**, available from
Xynergy Products Ltd, tel: 0845 658 5858,
www.xynergy.co.uk

**Tweezerman**, tel: 020 7237 1007,
www.tweezerman.com

U **Ultraglow**, tel: 0800 146 615

 **Vaishaly Patel**, Vaishaly Clinic,
51 Paddington Street, London,
W1U 4HR, tel: 020 7224 6088

**Valentine Alexander**, Face Focus; to book
a session, tel: 0795 684 6909

**Veet**, tel: 0845 769 7079, www.veet.co.uk

**Vichy**, tel: 0800 169 6193, www.vichy.com

W **Weleda**, tel: 0115 944 8222,
www.weleda.co.uk

Y **Yves Saint Laurent**,
tel: 01444 255 700, www.ysl.com

 **ZO1**, tel: 01753 759 746,
www.zo-1.com

# ACKNOWLEDGEMENTS

First of all, as ever, we send love and thanks to our agent Kay McCauley and to Kyle Cathie, the publisher who trusted our instinct with the first *Beauty Bible* – nearly ten years ago. Also to Kyle's entire team, particularly Julia Barder and Ana Sampson.

This book was 'turned round' as speedily as a magazine and the credit here goes to our wonderfully talented and efficient designer Jenny Semple, and also to our gimlet-eyed copy editor Simon Canney – both endlessly collaborative and unflappable.

We're particularly delighted with the shopping tips at the beginning and would like to thank Lorna McKay of QVC, make-up artist extraordinaire Jenny Jordan, superhairstylist Kerry Warn and nail technician Leighton Denny for their generous input.

Finally, additional thanks to Sue Peart and Catherine Fenton of YOU Magazine for their unstinting support and interest.

# DEDICATION

This book is dedicated to the tireless Rhian Hepple, Jessie Lawrence, Lily Evans and Elizabeth Guy for the huge amounts of hard work they put into helping us – and the endless hours spent in the 'Beauty Dungeon', packing up parcels to send to our testers! Also to David Edmunds – for wheeling the parcels down the road – and to Nicki at Hastings Old Town Post Office, in Butler's Emporium, who frequently couldn't move for sacks of lotions and potions, and to Margaret Sams, who tirelessly opened the door to couriers.

We'd also like to thank all the testers who diligently tested the products – over 2,400 of you, in all – and reported back to us, and the hundreds of beauty PRs who efficiently submitted their products for testing. Without all of you, this book wouldn't exist.

First published in Great Britain in 2005 by
Kyle Cathie Limited
122 Arlington Road
London NW1 7HP
www.kylecathie.com

www.beautybible.com

2 4 6 8 10 9 7 5 3 1

ISBN 1 85626 619 2

Text © 2005 Josephine Fairley and Sarah Stacey
Illustrations © 2005 David Downton
Layout © 2005 Kyle Cathie Limited

Design: Jenny Semple
Editor: Simon Canney
Production: Sha Huxtable and Alice Holloway

A Cataloguing in Publication record for this
title is available from the British Library

Colour reproduction by Scanhouse Pty Ltd
Printed and bound in Slovenia by MKT PRINT d.d.